NeuroAnalysis

T0221206

NeuroAnalysis investigates using the neural network and neural computation models to bridge the divide between psychology, psychoanalysis, and neuroscience when diagnosing mental health disorders and prescribing treatment.

Avi Peled builds on Freud's early attempts to explain the neural basis of mental health by introducing neural computation as a bridging science to explain psychiatric disorders. Peled describes the brain as a complex system of interconnected units and goes on to suggest that conscious experience, feelings, and mood are emergent properties arising from these complex organizations. This model describes mental health disorders in terms of perturbation to the optimal brain organization, and demonstrates how particular disorders can be identified through a specific breakdown pattern of the brain's organization.

This fresh approach to the diagnosis of psychiatric disorders will interest students, professors, and researchers of psychoanalysis, neuroscience, and their related fields.

Avi Peled is a psychiatrist with over fifteen years' experience of working with patients. He is currently chair of the rehabilitation department at Shaar Menashe Mental Health Center, and lecturer and neuroscience researcher at the Technion, Israel Institute of Technology.

NeuroAnalysis

Bridging the gap between
neuroscience, psychoanalysis,
and psychiatry

Avi Peled

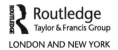
Routledge
Taylor & Francis Group

LONDON AND NEW YORK

First published 2008
by Routledge
2 Park Square, Milton Park, Abingdon, Oxon OX14 4RN

Simultaneously published in the USA and Canada
by Routledge
605 Third Avenue, New York, NY 10017

*Routledge is an imprint of the Taylor & Francis Group,
an Informa business*

© 2008 Avi Peled

Typeset in Times New Roman by
RefineCatch Limited, Bungay, Suffolk

Paperback cover design by Lisa Dynan

British Library Cataloguing in Publication Data
A catalogue record for this book is available from the British Library

Library of Congress Cataloging in Publication Data
Peled, Avi, 1959–
  NeuroAnalysis: bridging the gap between neuroscience,
psychoanalysis, and psychiatry/ Avi Peled.
    p. cm.
  Includes bibliographical references and index.
  ISBN 978–0–415–45132–1 (hardback) – ISBN 978–0–415–
45133–8 (pbk.) 1. Neuropsychiatry. 2. Computational neuroscience.
3. Neural networks (Neurobiology) I. Title. II. Title: Neuro analysis.
  [DNLM: 1. Mental Disorders–diagnosis. 2. Computational Biology.
3. Neuropsychology. WM 141 P381n 2008]
  RC341.P45 2008
  616.8–dc22   2007051692

ISBN: 978–0–415–45132–1 (hbk)
ISBN: 978–0–415–45133–8 (pbk)

DOI: 10.4324/9780203894736

If Freud was living today NeuroAnalysis is what he might have been writing, it is the missing link between psychology and neurology that he has aspired to in his initial endeavour in "The Project for a Psychology."

Avi Peled 2006

Contents

Illustrations

Acknowledgments

Acknowledgment goes to Rena Kurs from the Medical Library at Lev-Hasharon Mental Health Center for help in reviewing and editing the book. Acknowledgment also goes to my patients who have inspired me in this project and their clinical problems have motivated the ideas in this book.

Chapter 1

Introduction

Author's introduction

At the annual meeting of the Rapaport-Klein study group held at Austen Riggs Center in 2006, David D. Olds presented a paper on "Interdisciplinary studies and our practice." In his presentation he discussed the influence of neighboring disciplines on psychoanalysis.

Among other topics, he discussed "bridging theories" which may be traced back to the biological theories of Freud's Project (Freud 1953 [1900]: 536). He argued that the purpose of these theories was to provide a scientific basis for psychoanalysis. In today's era of "evidence-based treatments" this foundation could be relevant to measures of efficacy and thus may extend the cultural foundation for psychoanalysis. In my mind, most importantly, bridging psycho-analysis and neuroscience opens up each discipline to the fruitful advances of the other, substantially increasing our understanding of the human experience.

Even though they did not use the language of biology, psycho-analysts have developed a true understanding of the workings of the psychological brain. Recently, neuroscience, with the advance-ment of systems theories, is beginning to present evidence that may validate many psychoanalytic intuitions. Bringing these disciplines together may have a phase-transition effect on our understanding of the brain, which could potentially advance psychiatry towards the goal of finding effective cures.

It has been stated that we are at the phase in psychiatry where "astronomy was before Copernicus and biology before Darwin" (Kendell and Jablensky 2003). Combining psychoanalysis and com-putational neuroscience may lead to the "Copernicus Darwin effect" of phase transition we are waiting for. To date, any attempt to link brain neural activity and psychodynamic concepts requires a tremendous conceptual leap, which would be facilitated by developing a common language between brain and mind (Peled 2004). This monograph takes that leap.

Although we are dealing with an extremely complex field of research, due to the interdisciplinary character of the content, this monograph is intentionally written in terms comprehensible to the layperson. The neuroscientist may be a layperson in psychoanalysis, and vice versa. In addition, since a combined psychoanalysis-computational-neuroscience discipline is inevitably a discipline of the future, this monograph is also addressed to future generations.

I do not aspire to present a comprehensive review of computational neuroscience or psychoanalysis, but rather the bare basics of each discipline, hoping that this text will stimulate the reader to seek further information. For more extensive and in-depth information the reader is referred to the vast literature of each field.

General introduction

Freud and his successors (in developing psychology) have left us the unfinished task of relating their work to the functions of the brain. This is evident in Freud's writings. Freud was aware that some day a neurophysiological basis would be established for his psychological insights (Freud 1953 [1900]: 536).

In 1895, before he developed psychoanalysis, Freud attempted to explain the neural basis of psychological phenomena and disorders. This effort was formulated in a series of letters he wrote to his Berlin friend, Wilhelm Fliess. Freud soon abandoned his attempt to find an explicit neurological framework for his theories, probably realizing he was ahead of his time regarding neuroscience. Turning to develop psychoanalysis, as we know it today, he wrote:

> I shall entirely disregard the fact that the mental apparatus with which we are here concerned is also known to us in the form of an anatomical preparation, and I shall carefully avoid the temptation to determine psychical locality in any anatomical fashion. I shall remain on psychological ground.
>
> (Freud 1953 [1900]: 536)

What are the biological (neuroscientific) roots of psychoanalysis? To answer this question we need to go back to some of Freud's teachers who influenced the science of his era and thus the basis for psychoanalysis. We will refer to Ernest Brücke (1810–1892) and Theodor Meynert (1833–1892).

In a time when mental phenomena were treated in philosophical and religious domains Ernest Brücke stated that no other forces than the common physical-chemical ones are active within the organism. Thus psychic phenomena should be studied with physical mathematical methods. This trivial understanding of modern science had to be formulated back then in order to annex the study of the psyche to science. With this notion in mind Freud would later write to Fliess: "the intention is to furnish a psychology that shall be a natural science: that is, to represent psychical processes as quantitatively determinate stages of specifiable material particles" (Freud 1966: 295).

Brücke discussed a putative existence of an as yet undiscovered mechanism in the nervous system whose function is to "summate" excitation. Brücke suggested that excitation from the stimulus enters the nervous system via a receptor (meaning sensory organ), and then accumulates in a nervous center until a certain threshold is reached. Only then does the center initiate the reflex by discharging its accumulated excitation into the motor nerves.

Brücke's influence is reflected in Freud's letters to Fliess formulating a "Q" quantity. Neurons are conceptualized as receptacles that can be filled up, or *cathected* by varying amounts of Q. In this sense "catharsis" originated for describing what would today be called "action potential" of the neuron.

According to Meynert the cortex is the anatomical substrate of the mind with certain cells in the sensory and motor areas representing specific ideas and memories. The cells are potentially interconnected in a vast network by means of "association fibres," the bulk of whose substance lies in the frontal lobes. After two cells have been simultaneously excited (equivalent to simultaneous arousal or two ideas), an association fibre opens up between them. Meynert believed that a "train of thought" is simply the consequence of excitation flowing through a series of cortical cells that have been associated due to previous simultaneous excitations.

Each individual has a unique pattern of experience and so develops a unique pattern of cortical associations that represent his memories. These associations are the anatomical substrate of a person's "individuality," and Meynert referred to them collectively as the *ego* (German *Ich*). If the ego has not had time to develop, as in an infant, thought processes tend to be random or determined largely by any pattern of stimulation that happens to be effectual at a given moment.

Meynert also believed that the associations of an *adult* ego could be temporarily or permanently weakened, with a similar result of random or confused thought processes. The *sleep state* brings on temporary ego weakness, for example, with the consequent bizarre mentation that characterizes dreams. Toxic conditions in the brain can produce a more permanent ego weakness, resulting in psychotic states.

Thus it is evident that the term "ego" was pre-Freud and that Freud also shared the idea that activations of groups of neurons may represent psychological phenomena such as ideas and thoughts. In this regard Freud wrote that certain cortical neurons are the anatomical equivalents of ideas and memories. He called these neurons, collectively, the *Psi system* and formulated some sketch drawings showing possible "Q" energy flow from neurons representing "food in the kitchen" trying to draw the network representing the thought of going to the kitchen to have a meal.

Based on these early writings, one may assume that if Freud were living today he would be astute in modern neuroscience and might formulate psychoanalytic theories in terms of neuronal organizations of the brain, and perhaps even coin the term "neuroanalysis."

Today we can attempt to achieve Freud's initial goals by bridging the gap between his psychoanalytic intuitions and today's current advances in neuroscience. We can attempt to describe psychological psychodynamic formulations using insights from neuroscience and neural computation systems theories of the brain. To achieve that goal, a review of basic neuroscience and neural computation theories followed by the application of these insights to psychological formulations used in psychotherapy is in order.

This is not an easy task. While neuroscience and neural computation progress as scientific disciplines through the orderly evolution of empirically tested hypotheses and scientific experiments, psychoanalysis is a collection of suppositions based on clinical experience. It developed by refining and reframing the initial ideas of Freud and his early followers; thus it results in overlapping frames of reference that lack a universal orderly schema. To complicate the task, various psychoanalytic theorists use the same vocabulary but ascribe very different meanings to the terms, based on their unique orientations.

Although a comprehensive review of psychoanalysis and neural computation will not be presented given the multifaceted aspects of psychoanalysis, a reduction to presumably the most common conceptualizations in the field is called for in order to provide an adequate basis to pursue the goals of this project. The relevant points in each discipline will be discussed solely in the context of linking psychology and neuroscience. For more extensive and indepth discussions of the disciplines, the reader is referred to the vast literature of each field.

Emergent properties

Prior to embarking on the daunting task of relating psychology to the functions of the brain, a fundamental "psycho-physic" problem must be addressed. How can psychological phenomena be explained via physical biological events? The "materialistic" approach of "emergent properties" is suggested.

Emergent properties relate to synergism, "the whole is greater than the sum of its parts." Simply put, the characteristics of the system as a whole are not explainable based on the characteristics of its isolated parts. For example, in reference to our interest in mental functions as emergent properties of brain organization, in 1962 Rosenblat stated: "neurons have never been demonstrated to possess psychological functions (e.g., mood, awareness, intelligence). Such properties presumably emerge from the nervous system as a whole" (Rumelhart and McClelland 1986). It is evident from brain research that microcircuits of neurons possess more properties than those that may be deduced from our understanding of the single neuron (King 1991). Similarly, the properties of activated brain regions are greater than the properties of microcircuits of neurons.

Emergent properties originate from nonlinear systems. Nonlinear systems are those systems that have no one-to-one relation between input and output. In linear systems, the whole may be described as the sum of all its parts. A change in the total system obeys an equation of the same form as the equation for the change in its elements. Thus, linear systems cannot demonstrate more properties than those of their components. Nonlinear systems may result in responses (or properties) that are higher than predicted compared to linear estimations, thus achieving emergent properties.

In this work normal (healthy) mental functions are conceptualized as emergent properties of brain organization, and mental disorders presumably emerge from perturbed and disturbed brain organizations.

Chapter 2

Some psychoanalytic formulations

Ego, id, and superego

When Freud set out to develop a theory for motivation that would help explain human behavior and the formative elements that shape personality, he was largely influenced by his professional background and the science of his time. The laws of physics and thermodynamics were then developed, and Freud's biological and medical background (which included the teachings of Ernest Brücke) induced him to consider drives of biological energy that underlay mental phenomena. This biological physical notion asserts that each drive has four components: aim, source, impetus, and object. The aim is satisfaction and discharge of the instinct (eating for hunger); the source is a bodily need (i.e., physiological condition); impetus is the force of the drive, and object is the entity or condition that will satisfy the drive (Freud 1915a: 122–123).

Drives represent internal biological influences on human behavior. They are energy-driven sources of behavior; however, they are also conceptualized by Freud as ideas and thoughts. This additional conceptualization is probably the combined influence of Meynert's and Brücke's teachings. According to Brücke the neurons act according to energy forces and, according to Meynert, neuronal activations represent ideas and thought.

Working with hypnosis Freud realized that ideations and thought content can be unconscious. This is typically characteristic of post-hypnotic commands. Under hypnotic states subjects can be instructed to perform tasks once they are awakened from their hypnotic trance. The task is then performed but the subject cannot explain the reason for his actions. Such phenomena point to unconscious commands that are reflected in post-hypnotic behavior. Freud realized that conscious, unconscious, and subconscious events comprise components of our psychic (mental) system and may determine our behavior and thoughts (Freud 1915c).

With that realization the transformation of unconscious ideas and drives to conscious ideas and vice versa interested Freud, especially the manner in which unconscious motives influence thoughts and attitudes (Freud 1915b). Initially Freud placed more emphasis on bodily biological needs, instincts, and drives. Later on Freud also realized the importance of external influences (i.e., interaction with the environment). The need to mediate between the drives, their satisfaction, and the demands of the environment led to the conceptualization of the ego. The ego acts as a mediator between the needs from the environment and uncontrolled biological drives. The id represents the source for the drive energy. The id is unorganized where conflicting impulse and ideations coexist unconstrained by any organizing force.

Freud viewed the newborn infant as chiefly representing the id's masses of drives and impulses without an organizing pattern of activity and thus also without consciousness. The interactions and contact with the real world gradually organize portions of the id forming the beginning organizations which allow for consciousness to surface as the ego slowly emerges from these portions of organized activity. However, the ego is not synonymous with consciousness. Only a small portion of the ego is conscious at any given time. A great part of the ego is outside of awareness but can be readily called into awareness. This is called preconsciousness; however, other parts of the ego remain unconscious and not readily convertible into preconsciousness or consciousness.

The disorganized activity of the id cannot directly become conscious; however, from time to time portions of the id can be expressed in the ego by becoming connected with memory traces of repressed experiences and thus participate in the formation of symptoms. Presumably, disorganized expressions within the ego underlie mental disturbances such as loosening of ideations and associations, inducing disorganized distorted experiences. Thus the expression of the id's unorganized and disordered activity underlies symptom formations and can be pre-detected via slips of the tongue, and in dreams when the id's content is more manifest.

Developmentally the id is present at birth and functions before the ego mediates the apparatus of the psyche. As the ego emerges, it faces the task of controlling or transforming the impulses of the id.

The ego makes use of various psychological mechanisms, especially repression, in the process of controlling instincts. Repression keeps unwanted impulses of the id from consciousness, and this fosters the ego's growth. In mediating between environmental experience and drives from the id the ego "protects" our conscious awareness from unwanted unpleasant contents neutralizing non-adaptive (with regard to environmental demands) drives, not allowing them to interfere with our adaptive experience.

The conception of the id and ego forms the "structural" model of the psyche; they are hypothetical constructs. We can refer to them when observing behavior, as they serve to explain actions and attitudes. This is also relevant to all other psychological formulations.

The ego develops gradually as the infant grows to adulthood. The development of the ego reflects the maturation of the mental psyche apparatus as it manifests in a more organized fashion. Through parental training and early childhood education, as the ego develops it incorporates cultural and social norms as parent images within the ego, which Freud called the superego.

The superego has a censoring and criticizing power. It incorporates the norms and standards of society, and also includes parental attitudes as well as the ideals and self-expectations of the person. Because it was created in early childhood and infancy the superego is mostly unconscious and thus unavailable for reality testing. Irrational self-blame and excessive harshness with one's own feelings and behavior is partly explained by the powers of the superego.

Freud viewed the ego as the great mediator. In an executive manner the ego acts to reconcile the id, the superego, and the outside world of events. The ego must allow the id to discharge energy but not to the extent that it damages the organization of the ego. In particular, the ego needs to mediate the conflicting forces of the id and the superego. A balance between appropriate interaction with the dynamic outer world should be maintained; thus the individual's attitudes and reactions will remain adaptable and reconciled with the external environment.

Neurologically the id is first expressed in infancy. The id is initially disorganized, as the extra-pyramidal motor system is undeveloped. Sensory experience has not been integrated and the infant, who is initially blind; and may initially not associate various experiences, when he begins to see objects. For example, the infant may see his own hand touching an object but may not yet experience the hand as being his own hand. Thus psychologically the infant experiences the world as chaotic, uncontrolled, and disorganized. As connections are made between and within neuronal systems, both experiences become organized and associated and the motor response gradually coordinates to become goal directed and response related.

Psychologically the character structure, according to Freud, results from sublimation and reaction formation. These are unconscious processes that bind the forces of the id in such a way that the ego accepts them, without jeopardizing relations with the outside world. The concept of "multiple constraints satisfactions," and the manner in which biological neuronal ensembles within the brain can achieve Freud's descriptions, will be explained later.

This description of character formation shifted the attention of many therapists from the drives and impulses as the causes of character disturbances, toward the more subtle complex interrelation of id, ego, superego, and environments which may generate character and problematic behavioral reactions.

In instinctual terms Freud described how the "libido" (sex drive) manifests in increasingly more organized ways. Freud named each developmental phase by the zone in the body where libidinal energy becomes manifest, and defined the "oral," "anal," "phallic," "latency," and "genital" phases. This reflects sexual maturity from a general pleasure of the autoerotic infant to focused object-directed sexual feelings.

Interestingly the infant's social connection with the environment centers on the mouth. Having not developed control over movements and sensations, crying is the only action and eating is the only pleasure the infant experiences. Thus it is biologically suitable to see the oral phase as neurologically guiding the psychological experience of the infant. This is a very passive psychological experience that explains why "oral" traits in descriptions of personality relate to the passive early childish traits of character.

Using these terms it is no surprise that the anal phase is attributed to controlling traits of character. Once motor and sphincter control develops, for the first time, the child gains control over his environment. He can also control others' feelings toward him by proper bowel control, frustrating or gratifying his parents over issues of hygiene. These developmental phases in early psychological formulations echo the development of the nervous system in its early stages. These libidinal developmental stages created the basis for understanding character in terms of drives and libidinal energies. However, later theoreticians developed alternative theoretical frameworks for understanding character, theories not directly related to instincts or drives. Jung described the introvert and extrovert psychological types. The introvert is absorbed in his inner world while the extrovert who turns outward is much less concerned with his private experience and much more interested in what goes on in the world. Both of these types are subdivided into "thinking," "feeling," and "sensation" types.

Another substantial shift in understanding character was presented by authors such as Fromm and Sullivan. Rather than relating character to libido and drives, Fromm emphasized assimilation and socialization. He believed that character types are the product of the interactions between children and parents. Having been raised in a specific home the child develops certain attitudes which, had he been brought up in a different type of home, he would not have developed. The attitude of expecting to receive may develop in a home where kindness and giving is dominant. In a home with an atmosphere of miserliness, anxiety, and suspicious attitudes, the child may be influenced by a "feeling of scarcity" and may well develop attitudes of clinging to what he or she has for fear that supplies may be limited.

The importance of character attitudes in relation to environmental demands is emphasized by Fromm in his "marketing personality" description of our culture, which is a character opportunistically oriented to market value. "I am as you desire me" (Fromm 1941). Sullivan describes a "self-system" for character formation and he describes a self-system configuration shaped by environmental approval. The self-system is built around, and incorporates, traits which have been met with approval by significant others especially in childhood (Sullivan 1953).

These variations of character formation which deviate from Freud's original mechanistic libidinal instinctual drives model later conform quite easily with object relation psychology, where the emphasis moves from within the biological system to interactions with the outer world of psychological events. This idea of experience-related development of the nervous system conforms to explanations presented in this monograph on how the nervous system accomplishes its characteristic organizations underlying psychological phenomena.

"Identification" is another psychological mechanism used by the ego. This mechanism enables representing relevant relations with meaningful others. With the identification of external objects (meaningful others) portions of the external world are taken into the ego and become an integral part of the internal world (Freud 1938).

The parts of the ego shaped by identification and internalization of relevant others (from the past) form a new psychic "structure" that Freud called the "superego." The superego has to do with early psychological relations; relations with the caregivers (i.e., the parents). Through education the parents help build a "superego" that represents the norms of society; thus morality and conscience are formed as controlling factors of the ego.

More complex representations are also incorporated as part of identification. In the "Oedipal conflict" identification of the male child with his father may direct him to loving and sexual wishes toward the mother (this is a part of identification with the father's affection for the mother). The conflict is inevitable as competition with the father is not possible. The conflict is resolved by repression and transformation but lays the ground for internal representations to guide later mature adult heterosexual attitudes.

Following Freud, later psychological formulations made by his pupils attributed broader meanings to the ego. The ego was considered "strong" if it effectively controlled drives, repressed frustration, and enhanced adaptability; thus impulsive individuals showing non-adaptive attitudes, victims of their instincts and drives, are often considered to have "ego weakness." In order to comprehend reality, "reality testing," ego functions need to include memory, thought, decision-making, and concentration. Thus cognition has also been related to ego functions (Fairbairn 1944).

There are two processes in the ego. In the unconscious primary process, thoughts are not coherently organized, feelings can shift, contradictions are not in conflict, and condensations (i.e., illogical mergers) appear; there is no logic and no time line. By contrast, in the conscious secondary process, strong boundaries are set and thoughts are coherently organized. Most conscious thoughts originate from this organized activity.

Id impulses are not appropriate for civilized society, so society coerces us to modify the pleasure principle in favor of the reality principle; that is, the requirements of the external world. The superego forms as the child grows and internalizes parental and societal standards. The superego consists of two structures: the conscience, which stores information about what is "bad" and what has been punished, and the ego ideal, which stores information about what is "good" and what one "should" do or be.

When anxiety becomes too overwhelming it is then the place of the ego to employ defense mechanisms to protect the individual.

Feelings of guilt, embarrassment, and shame often accompany feelings of anxiety. In the first definitive book on defense mechanisms, *The Ego and Mechanisms of Defense* (1936), Anna Freud introduced the concept of signal anxiety. She stated that it was "not directly a conflicted instinctual tension but a signal occurring in the ego of an anticipated instinctual tension." The signaling function of anxiety is thus seen as crucial, and biologically adapted to warn the organism of danger or a threat to its equilibrium. Anxiety is felt as an increase in physical or mental tension and the signal that the organism receives allows it to take defensive action toward the perceived danger.

In relation to mental disturbances it may be summarized that Freud considered the ego a generally dominant mental agency responsible for healthy mental capabilities, so long as it functions normally. Ego malfunction, in contrast, led to deep anxiety, and the weaker the ego the greater the anxiety. Thus, anxiety may be normal for infants and children, but is a signal of danger for adults.

Heinz Hartmann introduced the concepts of primary and secondary ego autonomy in 1939, and elaborated on them in later writings (Hartmann 1964). Within the framework of his description there is a conflict-free sphere of the ego. Hartmann focused on the autonomy of specific ego functions, and stressed that ego autonomy is relative, since both primary and secondary autonomous components can be drawn into conflict. He described and emphasized that the ego apparatuses of perception, object comprehension, intention, thinking, and language capacity are all congenital, and are influenced by maturation and learning. However, they are not derived from and are not developmentally dependent on conflict. Even so, these structures of primary autonomy can become caught up in conflict, resulting in inhibition of their functioning.

In secondary autonomy processes, attitudes that are initially associated with a conflict between drive manifestations and defenses can become detached from their sources. Both the stability of secondarily autonomous functions and ego strengths can be defined by the capacity of the various ego functions to withstand regression in the face of a focal conflict. Insufficient secondary autonomy increases vulnerability to ego regression.

David Rapaport (1967a [1951], 1967b [1958]) saw a reciprocal relationship between the ego's autonomy from the drives on the one hand, and from the environment on the other. Autonomy from the drives is insured by reality-related autonomous apparatuses and from the environment by endogenous drives.

Development

The developmental ideas around drives and impulses were preliminarily preceded by the idea of the "Oedipus complex." In *The Interpretation of Dreams* Freud explains: "It is as though a sexual preference were making itself felt at an early age: as though boys regarded their fathers and girls their mothers as rivals in love, whose elimination could not fail to be to their advantage" (Freud 1900: 256), and

> it is the fate of all of us, perhaps, to direct our first sexual impulse towards our mother and our first hatred and our first murderous wish against our father. Our dreams convince us that this is so. King Oedipus, who slew his father Laïus and married his mother Jocasta, merely shows us the fulfillment of our own childhood wishes.
>
> (Freud 1900: 262)

In *The Infantile Genital Organization*, Freud (1923e) described a complete reorganization, occurring roughly between the ages of 3 and 5, centered on the primacy of the penis as an erotogenic zone and on the Oedipal drama. "stages" or "phases," also referred to as "organizations," are each characterized by the primacy of a particular erotogenic zone. Thus, the oral phase is followed by the anal, the phallic (or Oedipal), and then, after a "period of latency," adult genital organization. The phallic phase is the high point of the oedipal scenario. During this phase sexual desires are directed toward the parent of the opposite sex, and castration anxieties, aroused by the child's fear of retribution from the rival parent, are most intense.

Later this conflict fades, due to repression, and the child enters latency. Puberty reactivates the earlier conflict in a new guise, but after Oedipal conflict equilibrium is achieved thanks to the onset of adult genital organization, there is shift of desire to a woman other than the mother, or a man other than the father.

Thus Freud developed a notion of development through phases; each phase was related to libidinal energy invested in biological aspects of the body, the oral phase, the anal phase, and the genital phase. In each phase a set of new, more advanced, psychological capacities are acquired by the developing human being. Other studies later developed this notion further. Erikson (1963) extended the idea of development to a full cycle of life from birth to death. While for Freud development is driven by energies of instincts (libidinal) from within the individual, for Erikson development is a series of crises emerging from the interaction of the individual with the demands of the environment, thus emphasizing the outer environment.

Erikson is most famous for his work in refining and expanding Freud's theory of stages. Development, he claimed, functions according to the "epigenetic principle." This principle says that we develop through a predetermined unfolding of our personalities in eight stages. Our progress through each stage is in part determined by our success, or lack of success, in all previous stages. Each stage involves certain developmental "tasks" that are psychosocial in nature. The child in grammar school, for example, has to learn to be industrious during that period of his or her life, and that industriousness is learned through the complex social interactions of school and family. The various tasks are referred to by two terms. The infant's task, for example, is called "trust–mistrust." At first, it might seem obvious that the infant must learn trust and not mistrust, but Erikson made it clear that there is a balance we must learn. Certainly, we need to learn mostly trust; but we also need to learn a little mistrust so as not to grow up to become gullible fools! Each stage also has a certain "optimal time."

If a stage is managed well, we carry away a certain "virtue" or psychosocial strength which will help us through the rest of the stages of our lives. On the other hand, if we don't do so well, we may develop maladaptations and malignancies, and endanger our future development. A malignancy is the worst of the two, and involves too little of the positive and too much of the negative aspects of the task, such as a person who cannot trust others. A maladaptation is not quite as bad and involves too much of the positive and too little of the negative, such as a person who is too trusting.

Phases are from I to VIII: I (age 0–1) infant, trust vs. mistrust. II (age 2–3) toddler, autonomy vs. shame and doubt. III (age 3–6) preschooler, initiative vs. guilt. IV (age 7–12) school-age child, industry vs. inferiority. V (age 12–18) adolescence, ego-identity vs. role-confusion. VI (the twenties) young adult, intimacy vs. isolation. VII (late twenties to fifties) middle adult, generativity vs. self-absorption. VIII (fifties and beyond) old adult, integrity vs. despair.

Thus, each stage can conclude in various profitable ways reaching a higher level of performance as new psychological capacities materialize, or conversely the crises may fail to resolve "damaging" specific developmental phases, leaving the individual with psychological deficits weakness and psychological sensitivity.

Defense mechanisms

For Freud, the concept of defense refers to the ego's transformation of painful, intolerable, or unacceptable ideas and processes into tolerable formations that would not harm the ego's organization. The concept of defense first appeared in his article "The neuro-psychoses of defense" and was next discussed in "Further remarks on the neuro-psychoses of defense," and "The aetiology of hysteria" (Freud 1953 [1900]). Finally, in the text entitled *Instincts and their Vicissitudes*, turning against the self and reversal into the opposite were identified as defense mechanisms, in addition to repression and sublimation (Freud 1936).

For a period, Freud abandoned the concept of defense in favor of the concept of repression. He then reintroduced it in "Neurotic mechanisms in jealousy, paranoia and homosexuality" (Freud 1923). Then in *Inhibitions, Symptoms and Anxiety* (Freud 1926 [1925]), he reconsidered this concept in relation to that of repression, suggesting that we employ it explicitly as a general designation for all the techniques the ego uses in conflicts which may lead to a neurosis. Freud thought that "further investigations may show that there is an intimate connection between special forms of defense and particular illnesses, as, for instance, between repression and hysteria."

Defense mechanisms are attributed to the organized ego. They maintain optimal psychic conditions in a way that helps the subject's ego both to confront and avoid anxiety and psychic disturbances. They are therefore directed toward working through psychic conflicts but if they are excessive or inappropriate they can disturb psychic growth.

Later, Heinz Hartmann (1950), in the context of his theory of the autonomous functions of the ego, argued that neurotic defense mechanisms constitute an exaggeration or a distortion of regulating and adaptive mechanisms. Anna Freud listed and described the ego's defense mechanisms. She identified "regression, repression, reaction-formation, isolation, undoing, projection, introjection, turning against the self and reversal," and suggested that "we must add a tenth, which pertains rather to the study of the normal than to that of neurosis: sublimation, or displacement of instinctual aims" (Anna Freud 1936: 47). For her, "every vicissitude to which the instincts are liable has its origin in some ego-activity." Without the intervention of the ego, every instinct would achieve "gratification" (Anna Freud 1936: 47).

According to the Kleinian School, defense mechanisms take a different form in a structured ego from that assumed in a primitive, unstructured ego. The defenses become modes of mental functioning. For Susan Isaacs (1952), all mental mechanisms are linked to fantasies, such as devouring, absorbing, or rejecting. Melanie Klein (1952, 1958) identified primitive defenses in terms of splitting, idealization, projective identification, and manic defenses.

As previously described, the ego develops with, and makes use of, defense mechanisms to enable mature organized conscious experience and reality testing. This allows for mature effective adaptive behaviors and attitudes of the developed adult personality.

According to early ego psychologists defensive mechanisms are typically unconscious "automatic," almost reflex processes. They are triggered into action whenever an unbearable anxiety-provoking ideation threatens to penetrate conscious awareness. Defense mechanisms work by distorting the id impulses into acceptable forms, or by unconscious blockage of these impulses. Defense mechanisms are healthy if used properly. Some disorders, such as personality disorders and psychoses, may in fact be caused in part by inadequate use of appropriate defense mechanisms. If misused, defense mechanisms may be unhealthy, i.e., when they become automatic and prevent individuals from realizing their true feelings and thoughts or when they put the person in actual danger.

Defense mechanisms can also be maladaptive when they are continually used in a manner that disrupts reality-testing. Repeated denial and paranoid projection can cause people to lose touch with the real world and their surroundings, and consequently isolate themselves and dwell in a world "created" of their own design.

As already explained, the first, and probably the most common defense mechanism is the "repression" of unwanted threatening drives and ideations. This is one way to avoid knowing or remembering, and thus experiencing unwanted content.

"Denial" is an ego defense mechanism that operates unconsciously to resolve emotional conflict, and to reduce anxiety by refusing to perceive the more unpleasant aspects of external reality. Denial eradicates unwanted contents from awareness. Anna Freud classified denial as a mechanism of the immature mind, because it conflicts with the ability to learn from and cope with reality. Denial can take many forms; denial of fact is avoiding a fact by lying. Denial of responsibility involves avoiding personal responsibility by blaming, minimizing, or justifying. Denial of impact involves avoiding thinking about or understanding the harm one's behavior has caused one's self or others. Denial of awareness is used to avoid pain and harm by initiating a different state of awareness; for example, with alcohol or drug intoxication.

"Projection" involves ascribing unwanted impulses to someone else, thus avoiding awareness of its content. In other words, projection attributes to others, one's own unacceptable or unwanted thoughts and emotions. Projection reduces anxiety by enabling the expression of the impulse or desire without allowing the ego to recognize it. A husband who may have desires of infidelity would become extremely jealous if he were to project these wishes on to his wife.

Dissociation is used in many forms. In psychoanalytic theory dissociation involves separation of a feeling that would normally accompany a situation or thought.

"Reaction formation" is a defense mechanism which involves doing or thinking the opposite; for example, a woman who is angry with her boss and goes out of her way to be kind and courteous. One of the hallmarks of reaction formation is excessive behavior. In essence reaction formation is the conversion of unconscious wishes or impulses that are perceived to be dangerous into their opposites.

Displacement is an unconscious defense mechanism whereby the mind redirects emotion from a "dangerous" object to a "safe" object. In psychoanalytic theory, displacement is a defense mechanism that shifts sexual or aggressive impulses to a more acceptable or less threatening target, redirecting emotion to a safer outlet. Displacement involves moving an unwanted impulse from one object to another, for example, feeling angry with the boss and wanting to confront him. This would be non-productive; thus transforming the impulse – quarreling with the wife – could be the result of displacement.

"Rationalization" involves finding a rational explanation for something you cannot admit. It is the process of constructing a logical justification for a decision that was originally arrived at through a different mental process. For example, your boyfriend breaks up with you and you rationalize that you never really liked him.

"Intellectualization" involves concentrating on the intellectual components of situations in order to distance oneself from the anxiety-provoking emotions associated with these situations. It involves turning feelings into thoughts. A person finds out that his partner has cancer, deals with it by becoming an absolute expert on cancer, and focuses on the disease intellectually rather than dealing with the emotions it prompts.

"Sublimation" is a defense that uses refocusing of psychic energy away from negative outlets to more positive ones. These drives which cannot find an outlet are rechanneled. In Freud's classic theory, erotic energy is only allowed limited expression due to repression, and much of the remainder of a given group's erotic energy is used to develop its culture and civilization. Freud considered this defense mechanism the most productive of those that he identified. Sublimation is the process of transforming libido into "socially useful" achievements.

Object relations

The body of literature that is typically related to "object relations psychology" emerges from various theorists. The multifaceted literature results in overlapping frames of reference that lack a consensus for an orderly schema. The reader is directed to the writings of Melanie Klein, Fairbairn, Winnicott, Edith Jacobson, Margaret Mahler, Otto Kernberg, and Heinz Kohut for an in-depth appreciation of this field. The following is a limited overview of object relations theory, concentrating on issues that serve as a link to neuroscience.

According to Freud, drives are directed toward objects, and pathologically, these objects sometimes become targets for gratification of instincts. The development of psychoanalysis after Freud has seen a shift of emphasis from the instinctual biological internal determinants of psychic experience to environmental or external influences that shape mental experiences. In this regard "objects" become important; they are related to meaningful others (i.e., persons) rather than to things, putting emphasis on interpersonal relationships. They are not only real objects in the environment; they are also internal psychic objects, i.e., they are the internal representations of real objects. Thus the individuals, who influenced our experience, are internally represented and as such continue to influence our experiences and the way we perceive our psychosocial world. The totality of our psychosocial perceptions, reactions, and adaptive capabilities is relevant to our personality; thus object relations theories are important constructs for explaining personality development and behaviors, as well as disorders of these human aspects.

Melanie Klein retained the instinctual basis conceptualized by Freud; for her the world of instincts is the world of fantasies which are the inner representations of bodily drives. Drives are directed to objects. Initially the ego is undeveloped and unable to perceive reality as a complex whole. That is why the infant can relate only to part objects, for example, the mother's breast. The relations with such early objects determine the first psychological experiences. If the object is gratifying (breast gives milk) then the psychological experience is good, and vice versa. Since the infant is undeveloped and the experience of self as distinct from objects has not yet evolved, then good objects mean that the infant is also good and vice versa.

Projections and introjections are mechanisms that Melanie Klein defined as related to the fantasy inner world of the infant. Projection is when the infant believes an object to be something from his inner fantasy and introjection is when something in the outer world is taken in, related to the self of the infant. Introjections build up an inner world that partly reflects the external world; projections of inner feelings color the infant's perceptions of the external world. Projection and introjection processes are especially dominant when there is no clear differentiation between self and objects, causing a bad object to generate a bad psychological experience of one's self.

A possible defense mechanism against the bad experience is "splitting" of bad representations from good ones. Since Melanie Klein believed that the ego is formed and develops via these mechanisms of continuous introjections and projections then bad experiences can "split" the ego, damaging its organizational development.

Regarding ego organization, Fairbairn (1944) wrote about the "endopsychic situation." He asserted that the ego seeks relationships with real, external people. If these relationships are satisfactory, the ego remains whole. Unsatisfying relationships, however, cause the establishment of inner compensating objects that actively fragment the ego's unity. Thus, the ego's frustrating relationships with objects become internal, and are active within the psyche, as if multiple egos are at war with one another.

Winnicott further stressed environmental influences by concentrating on the delicate balance between the environment and the evolving self of the infant (Michael 1986). The environment, when "good enough," facilitates the maturational processes of the infant. The infant depends on the provisions of the environment, and the environment (in the person of the mother, or primary care giver) adapts itself to the changing needs of the infant. The term "good enough mother" explains the need of the mother to adapt to the infant's needs. This adaptation causes the infant to feel omnipotent as the environment is recruited to his every need. Gradually pre-occupation with the mother is withdrawn as the infant grows, forcing him to see things more objectively. This transition from internal fantasy awareness to a realistic objective view of the world is a gradual process. Objects that have magical fantasy meanings gradually become real objectives, transiting through intermediate phases where the object is both internally subjective as well as externally objective. Winnicott coined the term "transitional object" which is typically a blanket or a piece of cloth that the baby touches and takes to sleep.

Kernberg described the formations of "structures" within the intrapsychic world of the individual. He referred to structures as enduring psychological patterns that result from the child's internalization of early relationships with people in the environment, principally with the mother. "Internalized object relations," as he called this process, are units that build the internal psychic structures (Kernberg 1978). Each unit is composed of three parts: an image of the object in the environment, an image of the self in interaction with the object, and a feeling that colors the object image and the self-image under the influence of whatever drive was present at the time of interaction. Simply put, the units of internalized object relations are a self-image, an object image, and a feeling or affect disposition linking the two images.

According to Kernberg the psychic structures such as ego and superego are gradually developed from internalized objects. If experiences are good, these good representations form "islands" around which the ego develops and grows. Bad experiences are split off as defenses of the positive experiences; thus bad experiences have a potential to fragment and damage ego organizations. As the ego matures internalization becomes selective and only representations that are in accordance with the individual identity are internalized.

In terms of development Kernberg thought that representations are initially undifferentiated; thus self-representation and object representations are fused together psychologically, and consequently the infant does not distinguish himself from others. Gradually the self differentiates from the object. Experiences with the mother at the initial fused stage, both good and bad, cause a differentiation or split between good and bad representations. As self and object representations are still fused, bad experience with the object (i.e., mother) is also experienced as a bad sensation of the self, thus there is an early split of bad/good experiences of self as well as object. Psychologically, others are experienced as all good (idealization) or all bad (devaluation). At this stage the ability to see both good and bad aspects in the same individual is lacking. Others are either idealized or devaluated and there is no middle way. The same applies for the self. Since the self is fused with the object, when relations are with an idealized person, then the sense of self is also ideal and elated. When the person in a relationship is devaluated, then the sense of self is also of low esteem and worthlessness.

Maturity of the intrapsychic organizations is achieved only after the self completely differentiates from the object and the good and bad aspects within the self-image and the object representations are integrated. This allows for the individual to experience complete independence from relevant others and to be able to recognize complex representations where persons have both bad and good qualities and thus do not need to be idealized or devaluated.

Kernberg worked with patients who had problems with the development of intrapsychic structures. The self that was undifferentiated from the object caused them to experience symbiotic intense relationships of dependence and dominance, while split (non-integrated) bad–good representations caused them to oscillate between extreme idealizations with self-elations and devaluations with deep self-worthlessness and depressions. It is conceivable that due to such instability these patients have difficulty maintaining normal relationships and are thus impaired in social and occupational achievements. For Kernberg, psychotherapy for these persons involved maturization of these intrapsychic structures.

Kernberg described personality patterns that are so vulnerable to fragmentation and instability that they often show disintegration of psychic functions, similar to those of psychotic schizophrenia patients. These patients were called "borderline" because they function on the "border" of psychosis and could easily deteriorate into psychotic episodes.

Kohut worked with patients with narcissistic personality disorders. His formulations discuss the development of the "self" in relation to early significant relationships (Kohut 1971). He thought that these patients were unable to rely on their own inner resources and therefore created intense attachments with others. Kohut's theory describes how a rudimentary self emerges from relatedness with others in the environment, and then becomes a cohesive self. According to Kohut this process involves "transmuting internalizations" by which aspects of the self-object are absorbed into the child's self. Normal parents will occasionally fall short of or delay gratification of a child's needs, but the frustration is tolerable, not traumatic, and gratification is not overindulgent. This optimal frustration compels a child to accommodate aspects of the self-object in the form of specific functions. In this process the inner structure performs for the child some function previously performed by the object.

Self-esteem is initially grandiose as the child receives all the attention and gratification, and experiences the sensation that all his needs can be fulfilled just because they exist. Gradually with "non-traumatic failures" that occur in transmuting internalizations, the self becomes more realistic and integrates with the mature personality. Such maturation of the self supports the personality with self-esteem, ambitions, appreciation of the other, and the desire to be loved and to love another.

In cases where non-traumatic failures do not occur (e.g., over-protective mothers), or in cases of traumatic failures (e.g., mother not available for the child) the maturation of the self can be hampered, either leaving the individual unable to cope with frustration because no frustration was ever experienced, or respectively leaving the child "hungry" for the missing love and attendance never received. In both cases the virtues of self-esteem can be seriously damaged, in the former case with the need for extreme dependence and self-assurance from others, and in the latter case searching for approval and attention. Either way the individual remains vulnerable to criticism, rejection, and in need of external reassurances to feel confident. These patients develop depression and anxieties in situations where these needs are not met.

Perhaps the most important practical implication of object relations theory is the conception of identification as a series of internalization processes ranging from the earliest introjection to identification per se, to the development of complex identity formation. Each step includes the internalizing of both the self and object representations and their effective interactions under the conditions of different developmental levels.

In the transference of healthier patients with a well-consolidated ego identity, the diverse self-representations are relatively stable in their coherent mutual linkage. This fosters the relatively consistent projection on to the analyst of the object representation aspect of the enacted object relationship. In contrast, patients with severe identity diffusion lack such linkage of self-representations into an integrated self. They tend to alternate rapidly between projection of self and object representations in the transference, so that the analytic situation seems chaotic. Systematic interpretation of how the same internalized object relation is enacted again and again with rapid role reversals makes it possible to clarify the nature of the unconscious object relation, and the double splitting of (1) self-representation from object representation, and (2) good from bad persecutory object relations. This process promotes integration of the split representations which characterize the object relations of severe psychopathology.

Carl Rogers (1965) suggested that the best vantage point for understanding behavior is from an "internal frame of reference" of the individual himself. He called this frame of reference the "experiential field" that encompasses the private world of the individual. According to Rogers, "organismic evaluation" is the mechanism by which a "map" (i.e., the internal configuration) of the experiential field assesses the psychological events of everyday life (Rogers 1965). Although Rogers is a humanistic rather than an object relations psychologist, the idea of the internal "map" of reference resembles that of internal representations which govern our experiences.

Chapter 3

Some ideas from computational neuroscience

Brain organization

Historically, brain activity was formalized using a localized approach of brain centers, defining specific functions for segregated neuronal regions. Later the integrated approach argued against localized functions and evoked a non-localized approach of spread activation and functional connectivity across vast cortical regions.

Today, it is recognized that nervous systems facing complex environments must balance two seemingly opposing requirements. The need to quickly and reliably extract important features from sensory inputs and the need to generate coherent perceptual and cognitive states allowing an organism to respond to objects and events, which present a combination of numerous individual features. The need to extract important sensory features quickly and reliably is accomplished by functionally segregated (specialized) sets of neurons (e.g., those found in different cortical regions), and the need to generate coherent perceptual and cognitive states is accomplished by functional integration of the activities of specialized neurons via dynamic interactions (Tononi and Edelman 2000).

The mathematical concept of "neural complexity" (C_N) (Tononi *et al.* 1994) captures the important interplay between integration (i.e., functional connectivity) and segregation (i.e., functional specialization of distinct neural subsystems). C_N is low for systems whose components are characterized either by total independence or by total dependence. C_N is high for systems whose components show simultaneous evidence of independence in small subsets, and increasing dependence in subsets of increasing size. Different neural groups are functionally segregated if their activities tend to be statistically independent. Conversely, groups are functionally integrated if they show a high degree of statistical dependence. Functional segregation within a neural system is expressed in terms of the relative statistical independence of small subsets of the system, while functional integration is expressed in terms of significant deviations from this statistical independence (Tononi *et al.* 1994).

One general characteristic of high mental functions is their capacity to flexibly adapt to the necessary information-processing mechanisms. For example, working memory tasks involve shifting paradigms, and the examined subject is required to choose from a set of stimuli (cards) according to a guiding rule (the color, shape, or a specific number of stimuli). The choice is based on the feedback of "correct" or "incorrect" from the examiner. After a certain number of stimuli is presented to the subject, the examiner shifts categories and the subject is required to change (adapt to) and choose according to the new rule. Adaptive performance is measured as the capacity to flexibly process the changing conditions in the task environment.

For a system to adapt to the environment it must master a degree of flexibility to change according to the demands of the environment (Ditto and Pecora 1993). If the system is rigid and unchangeable, it will not have the ability to modify according to altered environmental conditions. If a certain degree of randomness is introduced into the system, then the system is more susceptible to change and will modify according to the changes in the environment. Once change occurs in the system, it needs to be maintained over time for as long as it serves its adaptive function. If the system is totally random (changes continuously), modifications cannot be maintained for long periods. The system, therefore, needs a certain degree of order that will maintain the acquired change.

It is clear that for optimal adaptability, the system must balance orderliness and randomness in its interaction with the environment. In neuronal terms, randomness involves segregation because segregated neuronal systems will act independently of each other demonstrating non-organized, random activity. Orderliness in neuronal terms involves integration because each neural system constrains the activity of its other related systems via integrative functional connections.

In order to adapt to the shifting paradigms required by high mental functions such as working memory it is likely that brain function requires integrative as well as segregative capabilities. As explained above, the balance between integrative and segregative functions in the brain is achieved when neural complexity is optimal. As early as

1881, Wernicke regarded the cerebral cortex as constituting, in its anatomical arrangement of fibers and cells, the organ of association (Wernike 1881). Wernike perceived a hierarchy of an even more complex arrangement of reflexes in the brain. With this formulation he preceded later insights of brain organizations achieved by studying sensory and motor brain functions.

According to Fuster, there is a hierarchy of perceptual memories that ranges from the sensorial concrete to the conceptually general (Fuster 1997). Information regarding elementary sensations resides at the bottom of the hierarchy. The abstract concepts that, although originally acquired by sensory experience, have gained independence in cognitive operations are at the top (Fuster 1995). This information process is most likely to develop, at least partially, by self-organization from the bottom up; that is, from sensory cortical areas toward areas of association. Memory networks, therefore, appear to be formed in the cortex by such processes as synchronous convergence and self-organization.

In the higher levels, the topography of information storage becomes obscure due to the wider distribution of memory networks, which link scattered domains of the association cortex, representing separate qualities that, however disparate, have been associated by experience. Because these higher memories are more diffuse than simple sensory memories, they are in some respects more robust. Only massive cortical damage leads to the inability to retrieve and use conceptual knowledge, the "loss of abstract attitude" described by Kurt Goldstein (Fuster 1997).

Similar to sensory information, motor information concerning planning and deciding has also been hierarchically described. As first suggested by Jackson (1969), the cortex of the frontal lobe computes the highest levels of motor information. The primary motor cortex is at the lowest cortical level and represents and mediates elementary motor performance. The pre-frontal cortex, conventionally considered the association cortex of the frontal lobe, represents the highest level of the motor hierarchy (Jackson 1969; Feinberg and Guazzelli 1999). This position signifies a role not only in the representation of complex actions (concepts of action, plans, and programs) but also in their enactment, including the working memory (Goldman-Rakic 1987). The pre-frontal cortex develops late, both phylogenetically and ontogenetically, and receives fiber connections from numerous subcortical structures, as well as from other areas of the neocortex (Perecman 1987; Weinberger 1987). This extensive connectivity links reciprocally the perceptual and conceptual information networks of the posterior cortex with pre-frontal motor networks, thus forming perceptual–motor associations at the highest level (Fuster 1997).

Mesulam (1998) reviewed brain organization leading from sensation to cognition. Unimodal association areas form part of the lower hierarchical organization; they encode basic features of sensation such as color, motion, and form. They process sensory experience such as objects, faces, word forms, spatial locations, and sound sequences. More heteromodal areas in the midtemporal cortex, Wernike's area, the hippocampal-entorhinal complex, and the posterior parietal cortex provide critical gateways for transforming perception into recognition, word formation into meaning, scenes and events into experiences, and spatial locations into targets for exploration. The transmodal, paralimbic and limbic cortices that bind multiple unimodal and the higher more heteromodal areas into distributed but integrated multimodal representations occupy the highest connectionist levels of the hierarchy. The transmodal systems with their complex functional interconnectivity actualize (see emergent properties above) the highest mental functions.

Via the various sensory systems, information is continuously sampled from the environment. Simultaneously the environment is subject to continuous manipulations by means of the motor systems. This cycle of continuous sampling and intervention in the environment is governed by the ever more complex circuits which characterize the hierarchical organization of the brain. This hierarchy enables the necessary associative transformations to support cognition that is typical of high mental functions, and that is heavily dependent on neuronal connectivity.

The transmodal connectionist level of brain organization plays an important role in shaping the characteristics of high mental functions. If, prior to establishing a connection, two neuronal systems could act independently one from another, once their activity is interdependent, the activity of one neural system or network will influence the activity of the other. This might explain the internal consistency we experience in our mental functions, and why reality is perceived as being coordinated audibly, visually, and tactically. Planning, thinking, and acting also have consistency; thoughts and reactions are goal-directed to the stimuli at hand, and match situational events. Finally, our entire conscious experience seems united in a single, complete, logical, and meaningful continuum.

Consciousness

Building on a "contrastive analysis" that compares conscious versus unconscious processes across numerous experimental domains, Baars (1988) presents an integrative theory of consciousness called the "Global Workspace" (GW) theory. Baars' theory is founded on the view that the brain is composed of many different parallel "processors" (or modules), each capable of performing some task on the symbolic representations that it receives as input. The modules are flexible in that they can combine to form new processors capable of performing novel tasks, and can decompose into smaller component processors. Baars treats the brain as a large group of separable "partial processors," very specialized systems that function at unconscious levels much of the time. At least some of these partial processes can take place at the conscious level when they organize to form "global processes." Global processes carry the conscious information and are formed from competing and cooperating partial processors (Baars 1988).

According to Baars, conscious awareness is subject to "internal consistency." This implies that multiple-constraint-satisfaction characterizes the interacting partial processors when they participate in the global process. This model of the brain is fairly well supported by evidence from brain studies (see above) and studies of patients with brain damage (Roland 1993). The model also complies with the notion that the brain is composed of interacting elements (i.e., information processors) and is multiply constrained.

To explain the differences between conscious and unconscious processes, Baars turns to the popular models of distributed-processing systems (i.e., neural network models (Herz *et al.* 1991)). Baars proposes that a similar structure exists in the human brain, and that it supports conscious experience. The structure, which he terms the global workspace, is accessible to most processors; thus most processors can potentially have their contents occupy the working memory. The global workspace can also "broadcast" its contents globally so that every processor receives or has access to the conscious content. Significant, though, is the idea that only one global process can be conscious at any one given moment. In other words, consciousness is a serial phenomenon even though its unconscious predeterminants are parallel processes.

Baars' important claim about consciousness is that it has internal consistency, a property not shared by the collection of unconscious processes in the brain. Baars cites as an example of this property the experience of viewing a Necker-cube, an optical illusion which we can consciously see in one of two different orientations. The two views of the cube can "flip" back and forth, but we cannot entertain both of them simultaneously. In other words, our conscious experience of the cube is consistent. A similar situation is found with ambiguous words. People seem to be capable of having but one meaning of a given word in mind at one time. There is evidence, though, that the alternative meanings are represented unconsciously in the brain at the same time as the conscious meaning, in that the other meanings of such words often show priming effects on sentence comprehension (Manschreck *et al.* 1988; Neely 1991). This indicates that, while conscious processes are consistent, the collections of unconscious processes are not.

To summarize, Baars postulated a theoretical workspace where global processes are formed from the interactions of many partial processes. He postulated that the global formations in the workspace carry the global dominant message of conscious awareness (Baars 1988). Partial processes are specialized processes, each processing its information in an independent fashion. They function in parallel and, if not involved in any global organization, they proceed disconnected from other processes. Partial processes compete, cooperate, and interact to gain access to and participate in global organizations. The global formation may be viewed as a complex network of partial processes.

In global formations there are internal consistencies; consequently multiple constraints are formed between partial processes. When partial processes participate in the organization of a global process they are constrained by the activity patterns of the global formations. Thus, partial processes can no longer function (i.e., process information) regardless of the message. Partial processes are fast, highly specialized, and aimed at handling specific types of information. They are, however, limited in the extent of the information they can process, and they lack the flexibility and adaptability acquired when many partial processes combine and cooperate. Global formations have the advantage of both the complexity and flexibility necessary for efficient and elaborate information processing.

Combining Baars' theory with notions about hierarchical organization of information (memories) in the brain (see above), it is reasonable to consider that lower level partial processes in the nervous system interact to form higher level neural global organizations.

In addition, the idea of internal consistency in global formations captures the basic notion of multiple constraint organization. It is assumed that the dynamic activity of partial processes demonstrates both hierarchical and multiple constraint organizations. For example, once the partial process forms part of the global organization it is interconnected with all the other processes (i.e., it is broadcast globally). Thus, it contributes to, or influences, the global organization by virtue of its connections, i.e., by exerting its output through the connections to the rest of the system. On the other hand, because it is a multiple constraint system, many other processes will constrain (through the connections) its activity. One may conclude that from the information-processing perspective, the information delivered by partial processes concurrently influences and is influenced by the global message.

Due to internal consistency, if the information structure (i.e., activation pattern) of the partial process "contradicts" (i.e., markedly differs from) the information being represented in the global formation, the partial process will have "difficulty" gaining access to (or fitting in with) the global process. This is due to the multiple constraints between the partial process and the global formation, which will not be satisfied in such a situation. As global formations are higher levels of organization (from the hierarchical perspective), by constraining partial processes which are most likely of lower levels, top-down control blocks access of partial processes to global formation (i.e., "repression"). Partial processes compete for access to global formation, creating the bottom-up procedure. Thus, a balance between bottom-up and top-down processes becomes crucial for the contents that reach global formations and consciousness.

Tononi and Edelman (2000) combine the above insights with other findings and formulate the concept of the "dynamic core." The dynamic core explains which neural processes underlie conscious experience. Tononi and Edelman conclude that a group of neurons can contribute directly to conscious experience only if it is part of a distributed functional cluster of high millisecond range integration as well as a highly differentiated complexity (i.e., the ability to choose from many different states). The dynamic core is a functional cluster of neurons in the sense that the participating neuronal groups are much more strongly interactive among themselves than with the rest of the brain. In addition, the dynamic core must also have high complexity in that its global activity patterns must be selected within less than a second out of a very large repertoire.

The dynamic core would typically include posterior cortico-thalamic regions involved in perceptual categorization interacting reentrantly with anterior regions involved in concept formation, value-related memory, and planning. The dynamic core is not restricted to an invariant set of brain regions; it continuously changes composition and patterns.

The formulation of the "dynamic core" as presented by Tononi and Edelman (2000) summarizes many of the ideas about consciousness and brain organization presented thus far. First, it incorporates the idea of global workspace as a globally distributed functional cluster of neuronal groups. Second, it refers to brain organization at the edge of chaos (balanced between orderliness and randomness) by introducing the idea of the simultaneous need for integration and differentiation within the dynamic core. Finally, the dynamic core refers to the transmodal connectionist systems at the highest levels of brain hierarchal organization pointing to the relevant formulations regarding memory and mental functions described by Fuster (1997) and Mesulam (1998).

Plasticity

The relevance of synaptic plasticity to the information processing of the brain was recognized as early as the beginning of the twentieth century. Cajal (1911) was one of the first to realize that information could be stored by modifying the connections between communicating nerve cells in order to form associations. Thus, acquisition and representation of information basically entail the modulation of synaptic contacts between nerve cells (Kandel 1991). Information is stored by facilitation and selective elimination of synaptic links between neuronal aggregates that represent discrete aspects of the environment. Memories are hence essentially associative; the information they contain is defined by neuronal relationships.

Hebb (1949) proposed that "two cells or systems that are repeatedly active at the same time will tend to become associated, so that activity in one facilitates activity in the other." This is called "the principle of synchronous convergence" (Fuster 1997). Through summation of temporally coincident inputs, neurons become associated with one another, such that they can substitute for one another in causing other cells to fire. Furthermore, connections between input and output neurons are strengthened by recurrent fibers and feedback. By these associative processes, cells become interconnected into functional units of memory, or Hebbian "cell assemblies."

Evidence for synaptic plasticity was presented as early as 1973 when a group of researchers published one of the first detailed reports on artificially induced modifications of synaptic strength (Bliss and Gardner-Medwin 1973). They found that the stimulation of certain neuronal fibers with high-frequency electrical pulses caused the synapses of these fibers to become measurably stronger (i.e., their capability to stimulate post-synaptic potentials increased) and to remain so for many weeks. Their observation, which they called long-term potentiation (LTP), was probably one of the first reports of synaptic plasticity.

One critical component of the induction of synaptic plasticity in virtually all experimental models is a change in post-synaptic (sometimes pre-synaptic) membrane potential, usually a depolarization. There are two other common features. First, Ca^{2+} typically plays an indispensable role in triggering synaptic change. The elevation of Ca^{2+} may arise via flux through membrane channels, release from intracellular stores, or both. Second, plasticity usually comes in two general forms: short-term plasticity which is dependent on post-translation modifications of existing proteins, and long-term plasticity which is dependent on gene expression and *de novo* protein synthesis.

Finally, it is increasingly apparent that for many experimental models a vital bridge between initial induction of plasticity and its maintenance over time is the activation of adenylyl cyclases and protein kinases A. One of the more studied mechanisms of regulating Ca^{2+} flux in synaptic transmission relates to the N-methyl-D-aspartate (NMDA) excitatory amino acid receptor. Over the years it has become apparent that many subcellular systems combine in a complicated way to regulate Ca^{2+} flux and levels, for example, the phosphoinositide system, G-protein systems, and the neuronal membrane currents (for a detailed explanation of the relevance of these systems to synaptic plasticity see Wickliffe and Warren 1997).

In a series of experiments with the marine snail *Aplysia*, Kandel (1989) demonstrated how synaptic connections can be permanently altered and strengthened by regulating learning from the environment. Kandel (1989) found structural changes in neuronal pathways and changes in the number of synapses related to learning processes in the *Aplysia*. Essentially LTP is the mechanism by which *Aplysia* learns from experience at the synaptic level, and the experience-dependent process then translates into structural, "hard-wire," alterations (Singer 1995).

In another series of experiments with monkeys, the map of the hand in the somatosensory cortex was determined by multiple electrode penetrations before and after one of the three nerves that enervate the hand was sectioned (Merzenich and Kaas 1982). Immediately following nerve section most of the cortical territory, which could previously be activated by the region of the hand, enervated by the afferent nerves, became unresponsive to somatic stimulation. In most monkeys, small islands within the unresponsive cortex slowly became responsive to somatic stimulation from neighboring regions. Over several weeks following the operation, the previously silent regions became responsive and topographically reorganized.

Studies of the primary visual cortex in mammals typically show experience-dependent activity (Kandel 1991; Singer 1995). The blockade of spontaneous retinal discharge prevents the segregation of the afferents from the two eyes into ocular dominance columns; this finding suggests that spontaneous activity may promote axon sorting. Ganglion cells in the developing retina engage in coherent oscillatory activity, which enables the use of synchronous activity as a means for identifying the origin and neighborhood relations of afferents. However, substantial fractions of neurons in the primary visual cortex, especially those in layers remote from thalamic input, develop feature-specific responses only if visual experience is available. Manipulating visual experience during a critical period of early development can modify visual cortical "maps" in these layers (Singer 1995).

The relevance of Hebbian synaptic plasticity to mental functions such as perception, memory, and language can be best understood via artificial neural network models.

Neural networks and neural computation

Neural network models are simplified simulations of biological neural networks spread in the brain. Units in the model are simplified representations of neurons (with input summation and threshold-dependent output). The units are richly interconnected to resemble the massive synaptic connectivity found in neural tissue. These models abstract from the complexity of individual neurons and the patterns of connectivity in exchange for analytic tractability. Independent of their use as brain models, they are being investigated as prototypes of new computer architectures. Some of the lessons learned from these models may be applied to the brain and to psychological phenomena (Rumelhart and McClelland 1986).

One of the relevant models is the class of feed-forward layered network with added feedback connections. In the feed-forward layered network architecture, information is coded as a pattern of activity in an input layer of the model neurons and is transformed by successive layers receiving converging synaptic inputs from preceding layers. Added feedback connections transform the architecture of the network to a fully interconnected structure also named for its inventor, the Hopfield network. In the Hopfield model, "learning" is achieved by adjusting (strengthening) connections between the units to strengthen certain activation patterns in the model (Hopfield 1982). Strengthening connections simulates synaptic plasticity and the Hebbian algorithm in the model allocates higher activity to the units that are more strongly connected. Input is presented to the model in the form of an initial pattern of unit activation distributed over all of the units. The units in the model are then left to interact with each other. Due to the predetermined strengthening of connections the model "tends" to activate the pattern which is closest in configuration to the input pattern.

The distance between the input pattern and the activated pattern is measured in terms of "hamming distance" which reflects the number of units with different activation values between the two patterns. In this manner, the Hopfield model achieves a computation of content-addressable memory activation. The pattern strengthened by connection encodes the memory, just as Hebbian dynamics probably determines learning in actual brains, and the input activates the relevant associated (nearest in hamming distance) memory, just as one memory is associated with its relevant correlated memory. The content-addressable computation has been successfully applied to pattern recognition extraction and detection of visual and other stimuli, thus simulating brain perception and perception-dependent memory activation (Rumelhart and McClelland 1986).

The physics of brain dynamics and optimization

Optimization is typically defined as the ability of a system to evolve in such a way as to approach a critical point and then maintain itself at that level. If a particular dynamic structure is optimal for the system, and the current configuration is too static, then the more changeable configuration will be more successful. If the system is currently too erratic, then the more static mutation will be selected. Thus, the system can adapt in both directions to converge on the optimal dynamic characteristics.

Christopher Langdon discussed the "edge of chaos" as the place where systems are at their optimal performance potential (Kauffman 1993). At the edge of chaos, there is a sublime balance between stability and instability. This sublimely balanced formation is the state where the system is at its optimum adaptation and where it can naturally approach the more changeable configuration as well as the more static mutation. This balance is important for optimal adaptation to external and internal events as well as for "best solution" configuration toward these events.

The ability of a system to optimize is related to the idea of complexity as well as connectivity. As mentioned above, if the elements of a system are disconnected from each other and act independently, the system will tend toward randomness and thus to the more erratic configurations. If connectivity is dominant and fixed, the more static "freezing" state will prevail. Thus, the connectivity patterns in the system are crucial to the optimization and complexity of the system.

"Multiple constraint satisfaction" is the type of organization that accounts for the interrelations among multiple units in a system. Once the activity of unit A influences the activity of unit B to which it is connected, the activity of unit B is constrained by unit A. This constraint depends on two factors: (1) the activity of unit A, and (2) the "strength" of the connection to unit B. The strength of the connection determines to what extent the activity in A constrains the activity in B. If the value of the connection strength between the units is large, the constraint of the activity in A on the activity in B is large. Conversely, if the strength of the connection is small, then the activity in B will be less constrained by the activity in A. In systems with numerous interconnected units, each unit simultaneously influences (i.e., constrains) several other units; thus the activity of each unit is a result of multiple parallel constraints. When the activity of a unit satisfies all the influences exerted on it by the other connected units it achieves multiple constraint satisfaction. If the activities of all the units in the system achieve multiple constraint satisfactions, then the system as a whole optimizes multiple constraint satisfaction.

In order to understand the dynamic activity of complex systems, one must first understand the physics of "state-space." Imagine a system formed from many elements. The arrangement of the elements in the system represents the "states" of the system. Each distinct arrangement in the system forms a different "state" for the system. If the elements are arranged randomly, all the states in the system are similar to each other. If the elements of the system can form many distinct patterns of arrangements, then the system has many possible states. If the system can form only one type of arrangement, then the system is represented by one state only. The "space" of a system is represented by all the possible states a system can assume. If the system constantly changes, it is called a "dynamic" system. In this case, the system changes its arrangement from one point in time to the next.

To visualize systems and their dynamics William Hamilton, the well-known physicist, and the mathematician Karl Jacob devised the concept of *state-space* necessary for describing dynamics in physical systems (Ditto and Pecora 1993). A dynamic system is generally defined by a configuration-space consisting of a "topological manifold."

A point on the configuration-space represents the state of the system at a given instant. Each point is a combination pattern in the activity of the elements (i.e., the arrangement of the elements). The configuration-space of the system is determined by all of the possible states that the system is capable of assuming (i.e., all the possible combinations in the activity of the elements). This configuration-space is sometimes called a "landscape." As the dynamic state of the system changes over time, the combinations in the activity of the elements change (i.e., the points on the space change). The dynamics of the system are described in terms of state-space as "movement" from one point to the next on the landscape, defining a trajectory, or curve, on the configuration space.

If the system "prefers" certain states (i.e., arrangements) over other states, it will tend to be "drawn" or "attracted" to form these states. Once certain states are preferred by the system, they form "attractors" (basins) in the topological surface (Herz *et al.* 1991). If a metaphorical ball were rolling on the surface (space) it would be easy to see that peaks represent "repellers" (i.e., those states the system tends to avoid) and basins represent attractors (i.e., those states the system tends to assume).

Using the state-space formulation in relation to Hebbian plasticity and together with insights from neural networks, a memory embedded in the Hopfield model forms an "attractor" on the space manifold of the model. The attractor represents the dynamic tendency of the system to activate the memory states just as a ball may roll toward a basin of a landscape. Thus, multiple attractor-formations in the space manifold of a system could provide for internal information embedded in that system. In other words, the manifold topography of a dynamic system could well simulate internal representations achieved by that system.

The internal representations in the brain probably follow the general rules of Hebbian plasticity. Since the brain operates on the border of chaos, balanced between orderliness and randomness, the internal representations are probably subject to continuously changing influences. A more complete characterization of the functional connectivity of the brain must therefore relate to the statistical structure of the signals sampled from the environment. Such signals activate specific neural populations and, as a result, synaptic connections between them are strengthened or weakened. In the course of development and experience, the fit or match between the functional connectivity of the brain and the statistical structure of signals sampled from the environment tends to increase progressively through processes of variation and selection mediated at the level of the synapses (Edelman 1987).

Tononi and colleagues introduced a statistical measure, called "matching complexity" (C_M), which reflects the change in C_N observed when a neural system receives sensory input (Tononi $et\ al.$ 1996). Through computer simulations, they showed that when the synaptic connectivity of a simplified cortical area is randomly organized, C_M is low and the functional connectivity does not fit the statistical structure of the sensory input. If, however, the synaptic connectivity is modified and the functional connectivity is altered so that many intrinsic correlations are strongly activated by the input, C_M increases. They also demonstrated that once a repertoire of intrinsic correlations has been selected which adaptively matches the statistical structure of the sensory input, that repertoire becomes critical to the way in which the brain categorizes individual stimuli (i.e., perceives stimuli).

Thus, the internal representations embedded as statistically input-matching patterns are continuously altered by the configuration of external influences. Once altered, the consecutive inputs are "interpreted" by the recently altered internal representations.

Nonlinearity and criticality

To conclude this section on computational neuroscience and the physics of the brain, nonlinearity as an inherent character of the brain must be briefly addressed. As mentioned above, nonlinear systems are those where relations between input and output do not have a one-to-one relationship. Nonlinear systems are often described by a sigmoid graph. The initial portion of the graph may be viewed as a "trigger-effect" in which a small increase in input results in a large response in the output. The last portion of the sigmoid graph may be viewed as "saturation-effect," since the increase in input levels does not increase the output further.

In physics, the point at which a system radically changes its behavior or structure, for instance, from solid to liquid, is critical. In standard critical phenomena there is a control parameter, which an experimenter can vary to obtain this radical change in behavior. In the case of melting, the control parameter is temperature. A self-organized critical phenomenon, by contrast, is exhibited by driven systems that reach a critical state by their intrinsic dynamics, independent of the value of any control parameter. The archetype of a self-organized critical system is a sand pile. Sand is slowly poured on to a surface, forming a pile. As the pile grows, avalanches occur which carry sand from the top to the bottom of the pile. At least in model systems, the slope of the pile becomes independent of the rate at which the system is driven by pouring sand. This is the (self-organized) critical slope.

Self-organization systems typically evolve through a set of phase transitions. In nonlinear systems bifurcation is a typical phenomenon of phase transition. The system driven to a critical optimal condition, when driven further by additional energy, becomes unstable and as a consequence forms one of two different organizations, each more stable than the prior critical condition. The term "bi (two) furcation" describes this tendency to form one of two organizations.

Generally, we can define criticality as a point where system properties change suddenly (e.g., where a matrix goes from non-percolating (disconnected) to percolating (connected) or vice versa). This is often regarded as a phase change; thus in critically interacting systems we expect step changes in properties and phase transitions in dynamics.

To conclude, criticality may involve both levels as well as patterns of organization in systems. As mentioned above, phase transitions going from one level of organization to another, the system may gain or lose emergent properties as per its transit to higher or lower levels of organization. For example, evolution is generally described as phases transiting from one level to a higher level of organization; thus systems of higher levels have additional properties as compared to the previous level system. Properties of a system can change abruptly according to the changes of organization patterns within the system. Nonlinear systems can react abruptly to small changes (trigger-effect) or remain stable in spite of large perturbations (saturation-effect).

Instability can occur in all kinds of structures from solids to gases, from animate to inanimate, from organic to inorganic, and from constitution to institution. External and internal disturbances can cause stable systems to become unstable, but this instability does not necessarily occur from some ordinary perturbation. It depends on the "type and magnitude of the perturbation as well as the susceptibility of the system" (Cambel 1993), which must be considered before the system is rendered unstable. Cambel adds that sometimes it takes more than one kind of disturbance for the system to transform into an unstable state.

Prigogine and Stengers discuss the "competition between stabilization through communication and instability through fluctuations. The outcome of that competition determines the threshold of stability" (Prigogine and Stengers 1984). In other words, the conditions must be ripe for upheaval to take place. We could superimpose this theory to many observable situations in areas such as disease, political unrest, or family and community dysfunction. In psychiatry it is especially appropriate to conceptualize the idea of acute reaction to stress and adjustment disorders. Cambel used the old adage that it may be the straw which broke the camel's back that finally allows the system to go haywire. This old saying reflects the idea of the trigger-effect bringing us back to instability as a "behavior" inherent to nonlinear systems.

Chapter 4

Attempting the conceptual leap

As emphasized by the title of this chapter, an attempt is made to link neuroscience and psychoanalysis. As such, this endeavor is preliminary, open to change, and to further development. As part of a conceptual linkage certain new terms that serve as interdisciplinary "bridge-concepts" are introduced.

Brain states and consciousness

Let us begin by relating to the organization of the brain as a whole system. Any referral to the brain organization as a whole system is inevitably very reductive; however, this reduction can be justified if it facilitates understanding the concepts presented in this monograph.

Let us use the physics formulation of state-space in dynamic systems. Thus we assume that the brain is an organization of many "brain units" (e.g., cortical regions, neuronal ensembles, cortical columns, and even single neurons). Each brain unit can participate in many activation states (i.e., active, partially active, non-active). Together, units can create countless patterns of activity within the "brain system." Each such pattern is a specific condition in the brain system; in other words, a "brain state." It is conceivable that the number of possible brain states that the system can assume is colossal (given only two activations, "active" or "non-active," two units can assume two states, three units nine states, four units sixteen states, and so on exponentially; the brain has approximately ten^{10} units).

Borrowing from the terminology of state-space formulations, let us call all of the possible brain states the "brain space." Since the brain is a dynamic system, as time progresses from one millisecond to the next, the brain state changes. Across time, changing brain states form a trajectory of brain activation, or a "brain trajectory."

If each unit acted independently without any relation to (or regardless of) the activity of other units, the entire brain system would be arbitrary; brain states would appear randomly and the brain trajectory would be random. But we know that this is not true for the brain. Brain architecture involves pathways, synapses, and connections among units. In effect the brain is highly connected to the extent that the activity of most units is constrained by (and constrains) the activity of the majority of the other units. Thus, brain states do not appear randomly and brain trajectory is not arbitrary.

Due to connectivity, brain units can unite, creating many brain states. These brain states can interconnect further, creating more dominant brain states from larger, more widespread, ensembles of brain states. The larger the connectivity the more integrated the brain states, to the extent that if all brain units participate in the brain state then that brain state becomes the "global brain state." However, it is conceivable that in a very large system not all brain states will be integrated all the time; some brain states will be relatively "independent" from others, in the sense that they will be less influenced (or constrained) by the other brain states. The brain probably balances equilibrium of connectivity where both large-scale integrations form together with smaller scale organizations. Thus connectivity and disconnectivity may be balanced to certain extents in the brain system.

Let us assume that one large-scale integration is always active in the brain and call it the "dominant brain state." Other, less dominant, organizations will be called "fractional states." Since dominant brain states involve large-scale activity patterns they can be conceptualized as "global processes" similar to those defined by Baars (1988). Since they form dynamics via connectivity which change in the millisecond range, they also fit the description of the "Dynamic Core" (Tononi and Edelman 2000). Both the global workspace theory and the formulation of the dynamic core relate to consciousness.

This is in accordance with the idea of emergent properties. Emergent properties arise from large-scale complex (nonlinear) integrations (or systems). Thus consciousness may be explained as the emergent property of dominant brain states. Our conscious experience has a streaming motion; we are conscious in time, aware of things as they are from second to second. This supports the idea of a "dominant brain trajectory" where dominant brain states are activated in a continuous sequence, just as our conscious awareness is continuous in time, as represented by consecutive conscious events that occur one after the other.

As mentioned above, not all brain units must participate in the dominant brain state; certain units can create fractional states. Fractional states are unconscious because they do not contribute to the dominant brain state. Their description is in accordance with the idea of "partial processes" described by Baars (1988). Baars argued that partial processes compete to gain access to global formations; thus unconscious contents of the partial processes become conscious when participating in the global formations. The dominant brain state is a dynamic formation of participating fractional brain states. One can imagine this as a pattern of cars on the highway. Traffic merges and branches out; however, the pattern of car flow on the highway is continuously maintained.

This description of the brain system and its dynamic organization is faithful to the model proposed by Freud regarding conscious and unconscious dynamics. Unconscious content can become conscious when fractional brain states integrate into dominant brain states, and vice versa. Conscious content can become unconscious when parts of the dominant state fraction away and are thus no longer part of the dominant organization.

As the interactions that create dominant brain states bind fractional brain states, and as these states are also formed from bindings of brain units, connectivity becomes an important factor determining the formation and nature of dominant brain states. As already mentioned, dominant brain states are not random and they therefore maintain a certain consistency. Consciousness is an ordered, consistent experience. This was emphasized by Baars who claimed that consciousness has internal consistency (Baars 1988). Such consistency is attributed to the dominant brain state preserved by the binding of units that result from connectivity in the brain.

The consistent character of conscious experience is related to the connectivity power of the brain system. However, our consciousness has many factors that need to be highly flexible; one needs to shift attention according to changing events or occurrences, and to rapidly adapt to new conditions. This requires flexibility from the dominant brain state. Flexibility is obtained if connections can be loosened and disconnected to allow for changes and new pattern formations. Thus the optimal condition for a dynamic changeable dominant brain state (adaptive flexible awareness) is a balance among a range of connectivity "powers" from overly connected to disconnected.

Disorganization of brain states and psychosis

Disconnectivity fractions the dominant brain state to the extent that it can become extinct. Over-connectivity may phase-lock the dominant brain state and freeze any dynamic change. In both cases consciousness is lost. This is supported by the knowledge that consciousness is lost when damage is inflicted on the highly connecting anatomical structures of the brain; the limbic, pre-frontal, and cortico-thalamic systems (Tononi and Edelman 2000). Consciousness is also lost in a generalized epileptic attack when many brain units are overly synchronized. Dominant brain states and trajectory should not to be taken for granted, and perturbation to these organizations may be caused by damage to the units, alteration of connectivity, and additional reasons that will be discussed below.

As mentioned in Chapter 1, Meynert described associations (connections) as the anatomical substrate of a person's "individuality." He referred to them collectively as the ego (Meynert 1968 [1885]). Accordingly, consistent patterns of brain organization as expressed in the dominant brain trajectory can be related to the concept of ego in ego psychology.

Adaptability, flexibility, psychological maturity and cognitive capabilities have been attributed to the ego; similarly dominant brain states involve the brain's computational neural networks that are responsible for human mental and cognitive capacities.

The ego develops from the id as a result of interaction with reality events. Brain organization is known to emerge through experience-dependent plasticity. The infant is born with a rudimentary nervous system where connectivity is not effectively established. Thus if any dominant brain trajectory forms it is most likely unstable and fractional. We know that experience-dependent plasticity defines Hebbian dynamics (see plasticity above) in the sense that consistent environmental stimuli repeatedly activate neuronal ensembles. This repetition strengthens connections in these neuronal ensembles, turning them to brain states that represent the relevant environmental stimuli.

If the id refers to a disorganized (random) brain trajectory, the ego refers to a balanced, consistent, and well-organized dominant brain trajectory. The process of the development of brain organization through repeated experiences gradually forms ever more complex brain organizations leading from an initially fractional unorganized brain to a highly organized complex brain. The highly organized brain supports the dominant brain trajectory, which enables the appearance of computational ability, reflected by a mature personality cognitively adaptable to the demands of reality.

If we examine the environment into which the infant is born we find that the family and primary care givers are most relevant. Good enough mother, a term coined by Winnicott refers to the structural consistent care provided by the mother with a schedule of feeding, washing, and attending to the infant. From a systems point of view it may be concluded that the environmental system is more organized than the brain system of the infant. This organization structures the brain, gradually increasing its organizational level, by the gradually forming input-dependent stimuli-related connectivity. Repeated stimuli continually activate relevant neuronal ensembles which, according to Hebbian dynamics, strengthens the connections among the units of the neural ensembles making them functionally structured and organized.

If we consider the idea of interacting systems (i.e., the environmental system and the brain system), and extend it to the entire life cycle, then as the infant grows his brain system becomes more organized and his environment system becomes less organized. As the child grows he needs to confront new environments of kindergarten and school, moving from the protected, structured environment of the family home to the less structured, more hazardous social environment outside the home. Thus an inverse graph may be traced where the brain system gradually increases organization levels and the environmental system decreases organization levels. According to this graph, between the ages of 18 and 21 there is a critical period with peak vulnerability to brain organization. At that age the brain is approaching a good but not maximum level of organization, and the environment system is already becoming disorganized as the young adult needs to make his way in the world, confronting tasks such as choosing a lifestyle and acquiring a profession. The highly organized brain acts to organize the environment as he creates a stable consistent environment.

From this rough simplistic description of interacting brain–environment organizational levels, during adolescence and young adulthood both are at their lowest levels. Before that age the environmental organization level is high and the brain organizational level is low. After that age the brain organizational level is high and vice versa. This description of system-interacting organizations is important to explain why many mental disorders appear in adolescence.

This type of systems approach to the vulnerability of the organiza-tion of the brain is typically overlooked when searching for the eti-ology of many mental disturbances that manifest during adolescence.

If the infant grows in a disturbed family where the organizational level of the family environment is low, he or she may suffer mental disturbances. It is not clear exactly how this happens. The interacting brain–environment model can shed light on this question. If an impaired low-organization brain reaches the critical period in an environment with a low organization level, it will be unable to function and achieve an organized life. This impaired brain can have fluctuations in organization levels susceptible to organizational breakdowns, which clinically manifest as symptoms and signs of mental disorders.

Freud, and others who followed him, described the psychological development in phases, each phase allowing for the development of a higher level with new psychological characteristics. This description is faithful to the nature of nonlinear dynamic systems. Since the brain is such a system it is not surprising that the psychological descriptions concord with the neurophysiology of the brain. In effect, nonlinear systems driven by energy to higher levels of organ-ization show a phenomenon of bifurcation, moving in phases each allowing two new patterns of activity. This description accords with the developmental phases described by Eriksson. In each phase suc-cess or failure can be achieved (bifurcation), success is associated with development of a new virtue, and failure with the acquisition of a certain insufficiency relevant to that phase. Many psychological theories and formulations discuss the importance of stability and good object relationships for a mature personality to develop. These theoreticians describe psychological development starting from rudi-mental preliminary organization that is typically fragmented and unstable, gradually developing into whole complex intrapsychic structures. For example, Melanie Klein notes the infant's ability to relate only to part objects, Kernberg talks about "islands" of internalized objects around which future structures will be organ-ized, and Kohut talks about the "rudimentary self" unintegrated into the identity of the individual. These authors all agree that good experiences enhance maturation and organization, and that bad experiences are split off from the organizing structures and ham-per the overall organization. Either as defense or as damaging phe-nomena, bad experiences destabilize and fragment the intrapsychic structures such as the ego.

As mentioned above, the dominant brain states and their trajectories have consistency and coherency due to the connectivity powers of the brain; thus it is conceivable that the brain states that comprise dominant brain organization need to show a certain degree of dependence and constraints among them. If experiences activate neuronal ensembles and similar experiences activate similar patterns of brain states, then activations would maintain dependence and constraints among themselves. However, if experiences differ radically and their correlated brain activations have patterns that are far removed from each other, dependence and constraints among these patterns may not take place, creating fragmentations of dominant brain states.

Bad early experiences may be viewed as part of an unstable, nonconsistent upbringing where the child's needs are inconsistently met and where experiences can differ largely due to these inconsistencies. Such events activate incoherent brain states, which have difficulty organizing into dominant brain states leaving the individual vulnerable to breakdowns in (and fragmentations of) the dominant brain states and trajectories.

If we consider that ego formation corresponds to dominant brain states formation then it is comprehensible that psychologically we are talking about ego weakness. In addition, fragmentation of brain states parallels disintegration of consciousness, allowing all types of pathological experiences to emerge. Disintegration of sensory modalities (e.g., auditory, visual) may be responsible for auditory hallucinations. Disintegration with false reconciliation may cause biased false interpretations of events with the emergence of delusions. These psychotic symptoms that arise in a weakened dominant brain trajectory are in concert with Kernberg's descriptions regarding borderline personality organization and with Meynert's early intuitions.

As mentioned in Chapter 1, Meynert believed that the associations of an adult ego could be temporarily or permanently weakened. He believed that certain conditions in the brain can produce ego weakness resulting in psychotic states. Thus seriously undeveloped and impaired psychological development could correlate with a severe collapse of brain organization (i.e., weakened associations, resulting in psychotic symptoms).

Meynert also mentioned that certain toxic conditions also weaken associations (i.e., ego or brain state organizations). An example is delirium that arises in demented patients from neuronal damage with instability of brain connectivity. This is also evident in toxic conditions caused by psychoactive drugs that interfere with brain neuronal connectivity and neurotransmitter activity. For example, LSD creates psychotic experiences by altering neurotransmitter activity.

Although the causes of schizophrenia psychosis are not clear, there is evidence pointing to the assumption that schizophrenia is also a disorder of brain neuronal connectivity, or a "disconnection syndrome" as described by Friston (in Friston and Frith 1995). Some of the early findings supporting a disconnection syndrome for schizophrenia psychosis are as follows. (1) Principal component analysis of PET data suggests that the normal inverse relationship between frontal and temporal activation on a verbal fluency task is disturbed (they show weak positive correlation). This finding may suggest disintegration between the two areas in schizophrenia patients (Frith *et al.* 1991). (2) Studies with Functional MRI replicate these findings (Yurgelun-Todd *et al.* 1995). (3) Subjects imagining another person talking activate left inferior and left temporal cortices (McGuire *et al.* 1995). Schizophrenia patients not suffering from hallucinations have the same activation pattern as normal subjects. Schizophrenia patients suffering from hallucinations show a reduction in activity of the left temporal cortex, despite normal activation of the left inferior frontal region (McGuire *et al.* 1993). (4) Phencyclidine (PCP) is a psychomimetic drug that induces schizophrenia-like symptoms (Allen and Young 1978). PCP is a potent inhibitor of N-methyl-D-aspartate (NMDA) glutamate receptors. Glutamate neurotransmission is the mainstay of the excitatory cortico–cortical interactions (Friston and Frith 1995). (5) Reduced EEG coherency between frontal and temporal electrodes is highly correlated with reality distortion symptoms in schizophrenia, suggesting disruption of fronto-temporal connectivity (Norman *et al.* 1997).

More recent findings that support the disconnection hypothesis involve EEG coherence task-locked to the delay-response epochs of a working memory test. Schizophrenia patients showed less coherent activity during the delay period of the working memory task (Peled 1999). Previous work with gamma-complexity also showed loosened cooperation in the anterior brain regions of schizophrenic patients (Saito *et al.* 1998) and in acute neuroleptic-naive first-episode schizophrenia patients. Dissociated complexity levels partially regressed, similar to premature brains at an earlier age, were found in schizophrenia patients during a study of the neurodevelopmental hypothesis of schizophrenia (Koukkou *et al.* 2000).

In summary it is assumed that psychosis results, or is an emergent property, from global disintegration of the dominant brain state and trajectory, as this neurosystem disconnection fragments conscious experience. The specific clinical patterns of psychosis relate to the different neuronal subsystems which are affected.

Disorganization of brain states and anxiety

Clinical experience proves that psychosis is frequently associated with intense anxiety. The borderline patient, the patient with delirium, and the psychotic schizophrenia patient all suffer anxiety during their psychotic experiences. This leads us to assume that the connectivity disturbances during connectivity breakdown may result in an emergent property that is clinically expressed as anxious feelings.

In order to analyze these emergent phenomena of anxiety we refer to the idea of constraints among brain units (and states) caused by connectivity as mentioned above. In a system, "connection" signifies constraint and the fact that different parts are not independent. The knowledge of one part allows the determination of features of the other parts. A gas where the position of any gas molecule is completely independent of the position of the other molecules is an example of disconnection leading to disorder and chaos. An example of connection leading to fixed order is a perfect crystal, where the position of a molecule is determined by the positions of the neighboring molecules to which it is bound.

"Multiple constraint satisfaction" accounts for the interrelations among multiple units in a system. If the value of the connection-strength between the brain units is substantial, then the constraint of the activity in one brain unit on the activity in the other brain unit is substantial. Conversely, if the strength of the connection is small, then the activity in a brain unit will be less constrained by the activity in the relevant brain unit. In the brain with numerous interconnected brain units, each brain unit simultaneously influences (i.e., constrains) several other brain units; thus the activity of each brain unit is a result of multiple parallel constraints.

When the activity of a brain unit satisfies the input exerted on it by the other connected brain units, it achieves multiple constraint satisfaction. If the activities of all the units in the system achieve multiple constraint satisfactions then the system as a whole optimizes multiple constraint satisfaction.

Whenever constraint satisfaction in the brain tends to be disturbed, "frustration" of the connection between the elements in the brain occurs. Frustration indicates that connections are only slightly unsatisfied and implies that the elements of the system act barely in "disagreement" with the multiple connections among them. The elements in such a system will change their states (i.e., values) in an attempt to reach full satisfaction of the constraints, and continue to change so long as frustration of constraints characterizes the system.

Since the brain is a dynamic system (Globus 1992), once connections are satisfied, the system has already changed and a new set of constraints needs satisfaction. As such, a certain degree of ongoing frustration is typical to the system of the dominant dynamic state. If the frustration of the constraints increases, the dynamic process of constraint satisfaction increases, causing the elements to change their states more abruptly. If the frustration of constraint increases even more, surpassing the dynamic ability of the elements to change their states, a "danger" of breakdown threatens the connections.

Since the dynamic dominant brain trajectory results from a massive connectivity structure, multiple constraint frustrations can "spread" over many connections in the brain system, and to some extent be "absorbed" by the interconnected structure of the entire system. This process of absorbing the frustrations of the constraints maintains the stability of the global integration within the dominant brain state.

It is suggested that whenever the degree of frustrations applied to the multiple connectivity of the system exceeds the level at which it can be absorbed, the system is "destabilized," and the risk of rupture to the connections becomes imminent. At this level of disturbance, elements in the system change rapidly in a "desperate" attempt to satisfy their connections. It is suggested that anxiety is the emergent property from this type of instability in the neural systems, especially in those neural systems that are involved in global formations such as transmodal processing systems of the dynamic dominant brain state.

This model can explain possible relations between conflicting ideas, actions or motivations and anxiety. Let us suppose that a population of neurons processes certain information assuming an activation pattern relevant to that information. During the information processing constraints among neuronal ensembles become satisfied toward the relevant information-dependent pattern of activity. Now imagine that another set of information is applied simultaneously to the system. However, the new information contradicts the original information, pushing the system to an opposing configuration in comparison to the original information patterns. The result is that units in the system are simultaneously constrained to "comply" with opposing patterns of activity. Opposing patterns of activated units disturb the process of constraint satisfaction that takes place in the system and causes augmented frustration to the constraint satisfaction processes among units in the system.

Assuming that anxiety is an emergent property of constraint frustration in the system, it is comprehensible that conflicting information processing increases the sensation of anxiety. Conflicting information processing involves experiencing opposing stimuli and confronting opposing actions in decision-making. In effect, our environment as well as our brain system is dynamically changing to provide continuous frustration of constraints in our brain system, thus allowing for a continuous physiological lifelong level of anxiety to characterize our psychic awareness.

Disorganization of brain states and depression

When frustration of constraint is prominent in the dominant brain state it interferes with the flexibility of the brain activations over time and the ability to adapt to the necessary processing of stimuli. We have already described that adaptation is related to "optimization" in dynamic systems. Optimization is typically defined as the ability of a system to evolve until it approaches a critical point and then to maintain itself at that point. If a particular dynamic structure is optimal for the system, and the current configuration is too static, then the more changeable configuration will be more successful. If the system is currently too changeable, then the more static mutation will be selected. Thus, the system can adapt in both directions to converge on the optimal dynamic characteristics.

In complex systems the dynamics of constraint satisfaction among the units is in continuous flux and can proceed in two directions: (1) optimization, when more constraints become satisfied over time; and (2) deoptimization, when fewer constraints are satisfied over time.

Previously, we assumed that the emergent property of anxiety results from constraint frustrations; now let us assume that depression is the emergent property whenever brain state dynamics is subjected to deoptimization.

Deoptimization shifts in the brain system could be triggered by the alterations of the neural substrate itself (i.e., neurohormonal and neurotransmitter activity). Probably the hormone or neurotransmitter directly alter the transfer functions of the neurons, or their connectivity patterns, and directly alter the space-state topology of the internal configurations. In this manner, configurations that were "normally" optimized could now be deoptimized, triggering a deoptimization shift that induces a depressed mood.

To support the idea of neural network alterations in mood disorders there is growing evidence in recent studies that antidepression treatment is actually related to plasticity and connectivity of neurons in hippocampal and pre-frontal brain regions (Laifenfeld et al. 2002; Coyle and Duman 2003; Manji et al. 2003). Recent research into depression has focused on the involvement of long-term intracellular processes, leading to abnormal neuronal plasticity in brains of depressed patients, and reversed by antidepressant treatment (Laifenfeld et al. 2002). There is growing evidence from neuroimaging and postmortem studies that severe mood disorders, which have traditionally been conceptualized as neurochemical disorders, are associated with impairments of structural plasticity and cellular resilience (Manji et al. 2003). Postmortem and brain-imaging studies have revealed structural changes and cell loss in cortico-limbic regions of the brain in bipolar disorder and major depression (Coyle and Duman 2003).

In extremely stressful events, such as grief, or calamity, the external constellation of life events changes dramatically. The change typically involves "loss" (certain regular patterns of incoming stimulations are lost), and these are the information patterns that represent the lost person or the lost factor. In other words, the loss of a significant figure or factor in one's life leaves the individual without the "regular" usual environmental inputs which that person or factor had generated. Certain configurations that were normally optimized by usual environmental inputs will now suffer the loss of the optimization dynamics and will be deoptimized. This deoptimization can be enhanced by loss of connecting spines and marked pruning of dendrite arbores. Widespread deoptimization of many internal representations could shift the dynamics of the dominant system trajectory toward deoptimization and trigger the emergent property of a depressed mood.

Brain organization and defense mechanisms

According to Freud, the ego makes use of an unconscious domain of mental activity (the id) into which undesirable drives and ideas are repressed. "Repression" has been described as the mental mechanism that "guards" the conscious awareness from the intrusion of inadequate and intolerable ideas or drives. Freud indicated that the intruding ideas and drives from the unconscious actually threaten ego integrity.

If we adopt formulations about consciousness by Baars (1988), then repression can be reconceptualized as the dynamics of participating as well as non-participating processes in the global formations that support conscious phenomena. Partial processes that do not gain access to the global process remain unconscious (i.e., repressed). In other words, those fractional brain states that do not become part of the dominant brain state are unconscious. That is, so long as they do not gain access (i.e., do not become part of the dominant brain state) they are repressed. Due to the multiple constraints that characterize dominant brain states, certain partial fractional brain states may encounter "difficulty" in accessing the global formations of dominant brain states. This is especially true if the partial processes carry information (i.e., an arrangement pattern) that is entirely removed from, or contradictory to, global messages inherent to dominant brain states. Based on these assumptions it is possible to conceive what type of information will be denied access to the global organization; it will be the contradictory and unfitting messages (i.e., the fractional brain states) that activate patterns dissimilar, or removed, from the activated patterns of the dominant brain states. In neuronal terms it will be the partial arrangement that does not satisfy the global constraints. In fact, Freud described the repressed contents as "conflicting" topics or unbearable ideas. Here, "unbearable" stands for the partial process that is removed from (i.e., "unfitting" to) the information pattern presented by the pattern of the global integration.

A fractional brain state that has an activation pattern that is largely removed from the patterns activated by the dominant brain state cannot be incorporated in the general message of that dominant state without damaging its internal consistency and integration and is therefore bound to be excluded. For example, to a mother of a newborn baby the idea of killing her baby is extremely contradictory to the normal loving and "caring state of mind" typical to a new mother. If inadequate fractional states somehow gain access to the dominant state of brain organization they are inclined to destabilize or even disrupt it. If many conflicting and disrupting processes gain access to the global dominant brain state, the whole activation pattern of the dominant brain state may be destroyed and the neural systems representing it (i.e., the relevant neural circuits) are bound to destabilize. Indeed, the types of thoughts which involve killing one's newborn baby often emerge in mentally disturbed patients. It is thus conceivable that in fact certain fractional brain states actually do threaten the integrity of dominant brain formations and the actual stability of the dominant brain state and trajectory. This description conforms to Freud's notion of ego integrity that is being threatened by repressed mental processes of conflicting ideas or drives.

Occasionally, inadequate fractional brain states may gain access to the dominant brain states and are "transformed" in order to accommodate the global activation pattern of the dominant brain state. For example, immoral ideation is contradictory to the dominating content of a moralistic conscious awareness. Transforming the wish to behave in an immoral way into moralistic ideation may accommodate the prevailing dominant brain state of a "puritanical message." This type of transformation is known in the psychoanalytic literature as "reaction-formation."

Another transformation of unbearable ideation is known as "isolation." Here, ideation is not excluded from awareness; only certain relevant parts of it are "neutralized." These are the parts that are incompatible with the rest of the conscious message (i.e., the global activation pattern of the dominant brain state). The fractional brain state is included in the conscious awareness emerging from the dominant brain state, only to the extent (i.e., it is isolated) that it is removed from certain contents of the conscious awareness. If isolation is not enough to satisfy the message of the global integration, then "dissociation" may occur and certain contents of awareness would be ignored or experienced as independent and unrelated (i.e., split off).

The "transformations" described above are necessary to "protect" the global formation of dominant brain states from being disrupted by contradicting fractional brain states. Therefore, it is conceivable that these transformations justify the term "defense mechanism." They protect the global formation of dominant brain states and prevent its destabilization. From the biological point of reference, this may translate into destabilization of the interrelations between groups of neurons, which presumably have direct neuropathological outcomes on transmitter–receptor activity.

Freud affirmed that defence mechanisms reduce anxiety. The conflicting information in the form of constraint frustrations within global dominant activation patterns of the brain states results in the emergent property of anxious sensations. Thus it is imaginable that defense mechanisms actually reduce such constraint frustrations by allowing only transformed activation patterns of fractional states to participate in the dominant brain state.

We can assume that if defense mechanisms are insufficient, there will be repeated perturbations to the constraint formations and that continuous constraint frustration may eventually push the brain dynamics toward deoptimization shifts. This may explain why anxiety and depression typically manifest together in many patients (i.e., deoptimization results in depressed mood; see above).

Brain organization of internal representations and personality

We have seen that the extensive psychological literature on "object relations" relates to internal representations of the real world embedded in the brain. It is evident that object relations psychologists concentrated on the study of the dynamics of internal presentations and their relevance to personality and personality disorders. Internal representations on the neural network level of brain tissue may be explained using the knowledge relevant to information storage in the brain, that of brain plasticity and Hebbian neuronal ensembles. Using the state-space formulation in relation to Hebbian plasticity together with insights from neural networks, a memory embedded in neuronal tissue (similar to a Hopfield model) forms an "attractor" on the space manifolds of the brain. The attractor represents the dynamic tendency of the brain to activate the memory states. Thus, multiple attractor formations in the dominant space manifold of a brain could provide for internal information embedded in that brain (i.e., the internal object relations). In other words, the manifold attractor-related topography of a dynamic brain system embodies the internal representations of object relations.

Since object relations psychology is relevant to the nature of personality and is useful for treating personality disorders let us examine personality in relation to internal representations. Personality traits are enduring patterns of perceiving, relating to, and thinking about the environment and oneself. They are exhibited in a wide range of social and personal contexts (Sadock and Sadock 2004). Specific configurations of internal representations have firsthand impact on personality traits. For example, internal representations regarding hygiene, punctuality, and precision are more pronounced for some individuals, while for other individuals other representations are prominent (e.g., vanity and pride). The first example is typical of individuals who give special importance to order and strive to achieve perfection. These individuals are often referred to as having "obsessive" personality traits. The second example is more typical of individuals who regard themselves as special and important. They are often referred to as having "narcissistic" personality traits.

But what shapes these internal representations and how do they mature in the developing brain? From the brief preliminary overview of the psychology related to object relations it is strongly suggested that early experiences shape critical first internal representations. Later on experience keeps shaping the way we view ourselves as well as others in the world around us; thus interaction with the environment is the shaping force that determines our internal object relations. This is in concert with modern knowledge about the brain; "experience-dependent plasticity" is actually a neuroscientific explanation for such transmutations. Hebbian processes can now explain internal contexts and information built into neuronal circuitry.

Psychologists have described the gradual, repetitive processes of internalizations that take place during the development of internal representations; for example, Kohut talks about transmuting internalizations via "non-traumatic failures" that eventually result in a mature "self" integrated into the personality and identity structure. Neuroscientists have described the processes of "matching complexity" in which stimuli gradually alter connectivity patterns (i.e., Hebbian plasticity) to match input-related (outer-world correspondent) activation patterns in the brain. If we accept the previously described idea, in which internal representations are expressed by attractor formations created by altered connectivity patterns of Hebbian plasticity, then we have the neuroscientific assumption that may explain how the brain forms internal object relations.

Personality assessment equals the assessment of internal representations. Unfolding the subjective experience of the patient and his or her perception of the world, especially of interpersonal experiences, allows for the reconstruction of his or her "internal map" of organismic evaluation. Once reconstructed this internal map of representations (object relations) is a powerful predictor of the modes of reactions and interactions that the patient will actualize. One could

easily predict what the patient with predominant internal representations of orderliness and hygiene will experience when confronted
with filth and dirt. Personality traits (i.e., emotional responses)
emerging from internal configurations of object relations play an
important role in the interplay between internal configurations and
their optimization dynamics triggered by external events.

A mismatch between the internal configuration and the statistical
structure of an input set that is coming from a psychosocial event
in the environment can deoptimize the relevant set of internal configurations. Thus, an individual reared to appreciate hygiene and
perfectionism will deoptimize these representations when presented
with a situation carrying the information of disarray and filth. It is
proposed that the combination of certain internal configurations
(or sensitivities of personality traits) with certain specifically significant situations (or stimuli) may create frustration of constraints,
deoptimization shifts that could trigger anxious depressive reactions
(i.e., emergent properties). In effect, certain types of depression
(e.g., dysthymia, mixed anxiety, and depression) have been typically
related to personality disorders in clinical experience.

In addition to the "structure," "features," and "content" of
internal representations, the levels of their development also warrant
assessment. We have seen from the descriptions of object relation
theoreticians that internal object relations develop gradually from
initially primitive, unorganized constructs that can be rudimentary,
split, and incomplete. Such internal representations of context or
reference allow for partial and opposing representations to "split"
awareness and experiences. For example, partial development of
internal representations can induce "all-or-nothing" experiences
(black and white attitudes) impeding complex realistic experiences
(variations of gray spectrum attitudes). This mode of experiencing
reality is non-adaptive due to the wide discrepancy (mismatch)
between what is perceived and what is real. In effect the most serious
personality disorders have undeveloped, rudimentary, and partial
internal representations, meaning that they have non-organized
primordial attractor landscapes within the brain space. This
emphasizes the importance of assessing not only the content or configurational map of brain organization but also the level of development of these internal organizations.

Lower organization levels of internal representations result in psychological attitudes and complaints, which have been called "borderline personality organization." Higher organization levels of internal

representations show representational content-relevant attitudes and complaints. Various levels of organizations on a spectrum of personality disturbances can be described.

Authors such as Kernberg and Kohut excelled in describing the consequences of rudimentary partial immature object relations on the behavior of severe personality disorders. If the internal representations cannot distinguish between representations of self in relation to others, then experiencing attitudes toward others and self becomes fused with intense self–object dependency (i.e., dependence of self-experience on experience toward others). For example if the person in the relationship is devaluated, then worthlessness and self-belittlement is experienced. Split incomplete representations limit experience to the split representations, causing the individual to be blind to a whole integrated reality, and to experience only partial extreme aspects of it (i.e., all-or-nothing, idealization-or-devaluation). This inability to integrate experience toward oneself and others is reflected in extreme unstable behaviors and attitudes, oscillating between idealization of others (and self) and devaluating others and feeling worthless.

These unstable oscillating attitudes translate to unstable relationships in work settings and family frameworks, causing incapacity to hold a job or career and to maintain family or social relationships. These dynamics constantly cause frustration in the constraints among activated brain states and deoptimization shifts in the dominant brain trajectory, accompanied by continuous experience (emergent properties) of anxiety and depression (i.e., dysthimia mixed anxiety and depression according to the DSM [Diagnostic and Statistical Manual of Mental Disorders] diagnostic system for psychiatry).

Psychotherapy: a therapy of brain organization

Individuals often seek psychotherapeutic treatment out of distress that originates from interpersonal relationships. Initially the relations with the therapist will repeat the same patterns of interpersonal relations that caused the distress. The skilled therapist identifies these malfunctioning interpersonal patterns and during therapy behaves in a manner that gradually changes the attitudes of the client so that he or she will be able to respond more appropriately to similar situations in the future. This therapeutic intervention is called a "correcting experience." Better coping in psychosocial situations reduces suffering and enables relief from symptoms. Psychodynamic therapy involves overcoming resistance, offering appropriate interpretations, and increasing insight into relevant aspects of interpersonal relations (Freud 1953 [1900]; Michael 1986).

According to the approach of constraint organization in the brain, the psychotherapeutic process may be described as a physical change that takes place in the brain of the client. Initially, the relations between the internal map of reference of the individual (i.e., internal representations) and some aspects of the psychosocial situations he or she encounters are incongruous. This incompatibility reaches the extent where perception and reaction to those psychosocial situations are distorted and interfere with the psychosocial functioning of the individual. The psychosocial dysfunction is generally accompanied by distress, which is typically expressed through symptoms of anxiety and depression.

The goal of the therapy is to reshape the internal representations to include the appropriate internal configurations for coping with the psychosocial situations at hand. Initially, the client perceives the therapist as a person from his or her past. This is because the client activates the attractor systems, which represent the person from the past. Since the therapist is not the same as the activated representation, a distorted perception of the therapist emerges. Due to this distortion an inappropriate behavioral reaction to the therapist (transference) occurs. Most probably, this distortion occurs with other interpersonal situations outside the therapeutic sessions. This indicates that there is a substantial mismatch between the internal representation and the psychosocial reality.

The therapist strives to enlarge the repertoire of representations of the individual to match many more different psychosocial situations. In other words, the psychotherapeutic process increases the neural complexity (C_N) in the brain of the client (see above). When the therapist reacts to the client in a novel manner, Hebbian mechanisms of plasticity will gradually create the new attractor systems necessary for the additional internal representations. In this manner, the therapist "shapes" the space-state topology of the brain to form new internal representations. The process probably involves actual changes in the functional connectivity of the neural systems involved, and as such it is a physical process in the brain.

The process described thus far is actually much more complex than the above description suggests. For example, due to a lack of representational systems, the interpretations offered by the therapist are denied many times and do not gain access to the global formation of dominant brain states (denial). These interpretations will never reach conscious levels (resistance in psychoanalytic terminology). The sets of inputs from the interpretation of the therapist simply do not satisfy the constraints of the global configuration (i.e., dominant brain state), thereby conflicting with the message in the global dominant brain state. Thus it has been correctly indicated that for an interpretation to succeed it must be delivered at the right time (i.e., when the individual is ready for it (Michael 1986)). There must be a certain constellation of the global dominant brain state (i.e., organization), which is favorable for including the new patterns of information proposed by the interpretation. The therapist first prepares the patient by repeated clarifications, confrontations, and other interpretations. This process changes the global formation of dominant brain states, "moving it slightly" toward the pattern that will be favorable for accepting the critical interpretation (i.e., the one that will induce the change).

Freud indicated the importance of overcoming resistance in psychotherapy (Freud 1953 [1900]). By gradually changing the global formation of dominant brain states to a favorable configuration, the therapy enables the incorporation of an interpretation and the therapist overcomes the resistance to that interpretation.

Repeating this process over and over again will eventually "reshape" the state-space of the brain and increase the complexity of internal representations, and thus the psychological repertoire of the individual. These changes transpire and are maintained by the experience-dependent plastic processes of the brain. It is probably the increase in neural complexity that improves psychosocial adaptability. In turn, psychosocial adaptability reduces the suffering that originates from conflicts of interpersonal relations.

The outcome of psychotherapy is relief of distress in interpersonal situations. It is achieved via the reduction of specific sensitivities of personality traits and the increase of flexibility and adaptability to changing psychosocial situations. Increase of flexibility and adaptability reduces constraint frustration and deoptimizations of dominant brain states, thus reducing the experience (emergent properties) of anxiety and depression.

Chapter 5

Implications for diagnosis of mental disorders

Many of the psychological formulations may be described using neural computation terminology and insights from system theories related to neuroscience. Anxiety and depression may be reconceptualized in terms of perturbations to the normal dynamics of connectivity balances. More specifically, anxiety may be reconceptualized as a disorder of constraint satisfaction, and depression as a disorder of optimization dynamics. In addition, a more severe connectivity breakdown, such as significant disconnection, can explain psychosis. Considering that most mental disorders may be classified to one of these domains (i.e., psychosis, depression mood, and anxiety) it is evident that the formulations described thus far may be extended to propose a novel outlook on psychiatric diagnoses.

The current psychiatric diagnostic system, the Diagnostic and Statistical Manual of Mental Disorders (DSM) (American Psychiatric Association 2000) has recently come under increasing criticism (Frances and Egger 1999; Kendell and Jablensky 2003). The DSM-defined syndromes fail to describe distinct classifiable entities. Despite research efforts, none of the DSM-defined syndromes correlate with any neurobiological phenotypic marker or gene that could have etiological relevance. The efficacy of medications cuts across the DSM-defined categories, as both anxiety disorders and depression respond to SSRIs (selective serotonin reuptake inhibitors). The Research Agenda for DSM-V cites: "Reification of DSM-IV entities, to the point that they are considered equivalent to disease, is more likely to obscure than to elucidate research findings." The Research Agenda for DSM-V calls for a "paradigm shift" in psychiatric diagnosis (Kupfer *et al.* 2005).

Schizophrenia

The greatest challenge for psychiatric diagnosticians may be to explain schizophrenia in terms of brain connectivity disturbances. Schizophrenia is a complex disease involving many patterns of clinical symptoms. It has been assumed that disturbances of connectivity involving the organization of the dominant brain states are at the basis of schizophrenia symptoms (Peled 2004). It is proposed that the concept of neural complexity described above can account for most if not all of schizophrenia pathology.

Normal mental functions and normal coherent integration of conscious experience rely on optimization of connectivity patterns and hierarchical organization of the brain as captured by the idea of neural complexity. Schizophrenia emerges when these brain organizations are perturbed to the extent that neural complexity is disrupted. Typically, schizophrenia emerges with a psychotic episode; thus the initial perturbation to brain organization is of the "disconnection type." The balance between orderliness and randomness is disrupted and there is a shift toward randomness. The elements in the system become loosely connected and neuronal group activity becomes statistically independent. This in itself reduces the optimization of connectivity dynamics allowing for a reduction in neural complexity.

Assuming that the system tends to stabilize and resume optimization of neural complexity, it is proposed that in the process of stabilizing the system there are shifts toward increasing connectivity dynamics. This is probably a compensatory move to balance the system; however, this swing of connectivity dynamics pushes the system toward the overly connected activity allowing for orderliness to prevail and "fixed" connectivity patterns to spread in the brain. Neural complexity stays low since optimization of connectivity dynamics is not achieved. Over-connection or fixated dynamics is characteristic of poverty schizophrenia and residual symptoms (Peled 1999). Since the brain system probably strives to optimize neural complexity, at this point a tendency toward randomness is favored, leaving the system prone to recurrent connectivity breakdown and psychosis. In an attempt to reinstate optimization of neural complexity, the brain system becomes unstable, "oscillating" between "excessive" orderliness and randomness. These oscillating dynamics are reflected in the clinical shifting between positive symptoms and negative symptoms during the course of schizophrenia (Andreasen and Olsen 1982).

Balanced connectivity is probably continuously regulated by neural systems that have widespread distribution and influence many cortical systems simultaneously. Catecholaminergic systems (e.g., the adrenergic, serotoninergic, or dopaminergic systems) are neural systems known to have regulatory effects as well as wide global cortical distribution. It has been repeatedly shown that the dopaminergic system is involved in schizophrenia (Snyder 1976; Goldman-Rakic 1987, 1994; Davis et al. 1991; Grace 1991; Andreasen 1997).

The original dopaminergic hypothesis for schizophrenia proposed that hyperactivity of dopamine transmission is responsible for schizophrenia. This hypothesis was supported by two principal observations: (1) the correlation between the antipsychotic potency of neuroleptics and their potency to block D_2 receptors; and (2) the psychotogenetic effect of amphetamine and other dopamine-enhancing drugs. The dopamine hypothesis formulated more than thirty years ago still lacks definitive experimental validation and must certainly be modified to account for the diversity of clinical syndromes in schizophrenia and also for the complexity of dopamine transmission in cortical and subcortical regions of the brain (Soares and Innis 1999).

More recently, a dynamic perspective of the dopamine hypothesis proposes that an imbalance between cortical and subcortical dopaminergic activities could have relevance to schizophrenia (Davis et al. 1991). Two formulations based on this imbalance have been proposed. According to the first formulation, negative symptoms of schizophrenia are related to decreased dopaminergic function in the cortex, whereas positive symptoms are associated with increased transmission in subcortical mesolimbic dopaminergic pathways (Davis et al. 1991). According to the second formulation, low basal levels of synaptic dopamine predispose to excessive phasic or burst release of dopamine (Grace 1991). In both formulations, negative symptoms of schizophrenia are associated with low dopamine function and positive symptoms with excessive dopamine transmission.

Dopaminergic pathways relevant to schizophrenia are predominantly those responsible for synaptic connections with pre-frontal and frontal neurons. Pre-frontal functions have been repeatedly cited as relevant to schizophrenia (Goldman-Rakic 1987, 1996; Winn 1994; Lewis 1995; Selemon et al. 1995; Stanley et al. 1995; McCarthy et al. 1996). Pre-frontal associations play an important integrative function for typical high mental functions such as those tasks requiring delay response and sequencing of goal-directed decision-making or planning (Mesulam 1998). An overall view of the dopaminergic interactions with the pre-frontal cortex suggests a neuronal circuit for "complexity regulation" relevant to pre-frontal integrative functions. Cortico-cortical connectivity both within the pre-frontal cortex and with other cortical regions is sustained by the activity of pyramidal neurons (Fuster 1995, 1997; Mesulam 1998; Lewis *et al.* 1999). It has been suggested that reverberating feedback activity in these networks is responsible for holding information online to execute goal-directed delayed-response tasks (Frith *et al.* 1991; Cohen *et al.* 1996; Goldman-Rakic 1996; Lewis *et al.* 1999). These reverberating networks are regulated by the combined excitatory and inhibitory influences on the input–output function of the pyramidal neuron. Direct excitatory influences are provided by dopaminergic synapses on the dendrites of the pyramidal cell. At the same time dopaminergic synapses also provide an inhibitory effect on the same pyramidal cells via indirect circuitry: the chandelier interneurons (Lewis *et al.* 1999). Thus, dopaminergic activity is unique in that it both increases and decreases the activity of the pyramidal neuron.

This characteristic enables the dopaminergic system to promote and maintain neural complexity for integrated cortico-cortical activity of the pre-frontal cortex. Overall dopaminergic activity optimizes neural complexity. Whenever inhibitory effects "threaten" to disintegrate (segregate) the associations sustained via the accommodated activity of pyramidal neurons, the dopaminergic excitatory synapses rebalance the dissociation by increasing the integrative pyramidal activity and vice versa, and reduced dopaminergic activity will "loosen up" over-integration and over-connectivity. According to this description, the dopaminergic system could function as an "optimizing surveillance" of neural complexity. Such function is necessary in view of possible perturbations to the level of neural complexity that takes place during regular information-processing activity (see constraint satisfaction above).

As mentioned in previous chapters, information processing requires both integration and segregation between neuronal assemblies. Segregation is needed to allow for flexibility and adaptation to new patterns of information and integration is needed to represent and preserve the acquired information in relatively stable activation patterns for the relevant neural networks (Tononi *et al.* 1994). The whole system functions best at the border between randomness (i.e., segregation) and orderliness (i.e., integration) (Ditto and Pecora, 1993). The complex information processing in the brain probably involves dynamic oscillations between integration and segregation during cognitive computations (Paulus *et al.* 1999). These oscillations risk reducing neural complexity by moving the system to disconnectivity or over-connectivity dynamics.

If the hypothesis regarding complexity optimization of the dopaminergic system is confirmed, descending cortical pathways may convey information about cortical levels of neural complexity to subcortical systems such as the ventral tegmental area (VTA) and mid-brain of the dopaminergic system. In other words, descending cortical pathways monitor online neural complexity levels of the cortex. Ascending pathways of the dopaminergic system from VTA and mid-brain may complete a feedback system to regulate and maintain cortical neural complexity. Whenever the "information-processing load" perturbs the level of cortical neural complexity, the perturbation is "picked up" by descending pathways that reach subcortical "pacemakers" which then induce increased dopaminergic activity to "reoptimize" neural complexity.

As described above, reduced neural complexity in schizophrenia may oscillate between over-connectivity and disconnectivity. Sequential organization strategy in a neurocognitive behavioral task performed by schizophrenic patients may support the idea of reduced neural complexity in schizophrenia (Paulus *et al.* 1999). Schizophrenic performance was characterized by oscillating episodes of predictability and unpredictability in a left–right choice task. In this task, subjects had to predict the random appearance of an object on one side of the screen. Intermittence in the task was described by transition between two different states of the system, one in which temporally stable organization governs the system while in the other, the system gradually "escapes" organization into random activity. Patients showed marked oscillations between randomness and orderliness (i.e., probable oscillations between disconnectivity and over-connectivity dynamics).

Although connectivity breakdown refers to both disconnectivity and over-connectivity within the disturbed neural complexity, it is intuitively easier to initially describe it as a disconnection syndrome. Connectivity may be disturbed between brain regions (e.g., the frontal and temporal regions (Frith *et al.* 1991)), and also within brain systems (e.g., within the neuronal networks of the temporal lobe). Within the temporal lobe, disturbance of connectivity may account for reduced activation in that cortical field even though its correlated frontal activation is maintained (McGuire *et al.* 1993). In word-fluency tasks, frontal and temporal regions need to work together to enable the coordination of symbolic word representations with motor speech output. If the constraints between these two regions are not satisfied, each one of these processes may proceed uncoordinated and "regardless" of the other, leading to disordered speech on one hand, and disturbed goal-directed (planned) conceptualization (i.e., thinking) on the other.

The left temporal cortex contains the networks that integrate the hearing of words with their higher level conceptual symbolic representations (Mesulam 1998). This temporal cortex plays an important role in associating the heard concepts with all other perceptual occurrences, and thus for forming the sensation of a coherent meaningful experience. A connectivity breakdown within these systems may account for auditory hallucinations due to disconnections of the auditory perception system from the entire coherent dynamic core spread to other cortical activations (e.g., the frontal networks which continue to be activated). Cortical processes responsible for hearing words continue to function regardless of (or disconnected from) auditory processing systems of speech recognition. Thus, regardless of the fact that sound does not activate the auditory senses, and that visual experience does not identify sound sources, voices can still be experienced (i.e., auditory hallucinations).

Perturbed connectivity dynamics of higher levels of associations such as between and within transmodal regions may set the conditions for the appearance of delusions. Conceptions and beliefs presumably form at the level of distributed associative processes responsible for abstract conceptualization (Fuster 1997; Mesulam 1998). These conceptions or beliefs have been typically defined as "schemata" or "context" referring to higher order cognitive structures that underlie all aspects of human knowledge and skill. They are the stored traces of earlier experiences that allow for rapid unconscious processing of redundant information.

False higher level neural network connections (Hoffman 1992) may allow for the formation of associations that were impossible (or "wrong") before regular connectivity constraints were violated. The appearance of such "pathological" associations presumably plays an important role in the formation of false beliefs (i.e., delusions) (Hoffman et al. 1994).

Sensory evidence (from information of sensory processes travelling up the hierarchy) usually "corrects" and regulates faulty associations (delusional belief schemas) by making them "comply" with (i.e., satisfy the constraints of) the real conditions in the environment. Connectivity breakdown between higher levels of the hierarchy and lower levels of sensory evaluation may curtail the "correction," and thus faulty ideational (i.e., delusional) concepts may persist although information may suggest otherwise (i.e., unshakable beliefs). A shift of connectivity balance toward exaggerated connectivity could play an important role in maintaining pathological "wrong" associations. Over-connectivity could cause the system to "resist" any influence of change to the overly connected delusional pattern, thus reducing adaptability (schemata update) to the environmental condition.

Studies with models of artificial neural networks show that fixed connectivity models (i.e., Hopfield network) (Hopfield 1982) "push" the system to assume fixed states (i.e., converge into attractor configurations) (Herz *et al.* 1991). The network tends to repeatedly assume the same states over and over again (Hoffman *et al.* 1996). When applied to semantic networks (Hinton 1981; Spitzer *et al.* 1993) this activity is representative of repeated activation of concepts that metaphorically resemble perseverative ideation (that is, a few repeated concepts), and simulates poverty of thought typical to negative symptoms of schizophrenia. It is suggested that one of the deficiencies relevant to negative schizophrenia is over-connectivity within the networks of speech and thought representations.

Imagine that the breakdown in connectivity engulfs extensive networks both within and between systems of the hierarchy. In this case, combinations of multiple symptoms may appear. If connectivity breakdown is prominent within multiple systems, the perception of sensations, construction of concepts, and planning of goal-oriented responses will all be affected. Loosening of associations, delusions, hallucinations, and disorganized behavior will mix in a grossly disorganized mental condition. In these conditions it may be difficult to assess symptoms such as delusions or hallucinations because they will be "fragmented" by the loosening of associations and "covered" by grossly disorganized behavior (Andreasen and Olsen 1982; Andreasen 1984). This symptomatic profile is in agreement with the description of disorganized schizophrenia (Liddle 1987).

Reality distortion and poverty schizophrenia are two additional entities in the classification of schizophrenia (Liddle 1987). Reality distortion is typically dominated by hallucinations and delusions. In these cases, multimodal, heteromodal, and their connections with transmodal networks are presumably affected (i.e., temporo-frontal connections: Mesulam 1998) causing top-down bottom-up imbalances. Thus, the contents of consciousness cannot be controlled, because input and output processes are not automatically supported by global formation of dominant brain states that organize them into larger structures to provide context. Lack of top-down dominant brain state alters the meaning of trivialities. Normally, the experience of significance is dependent on the perception of patterned wholes. When the "gestalts" are deficient, details attract attention. Because they are experienced as new, they often seem to evoke a sense of significance unrelated to general meaning. Attribution of meanings to unrelated events may emerge just because these events are temporally occurring. Other erroneous reconstructions also occur, allowing for endless false recombinations of conscious experiences resulting from the loss of global contextual top-down bottom-up balance.

Poverty symptoms presumably emerge from connectivity failure of the networks located at the highest levels of the hierarchy. These are the networks that connect sensation with action (Mesulam 1998). Relevant social occurrences or other incidents in the environment fail to activate actions and responses of high-level integration. This leaves the patient behaviorally and emotionally unresponsive to the psychosocial environment; volition is lessened and any socially motivated action is abolished. Hypo-frontality, indicating possible failure to activate higher level associations of sensation with action, has been correlated with poverty symptoms (Andreasen 1983).

Perturbation to connectivity dynamics could result from a multitude of etiologies that support the "stress-diathesis hypothesis" for schizophrenia (Sadock and Sadock 2004). Genetic to neurotransmitter alterations can lay the ground for the "diathesis" component of the model, and stressful events, typically of a conflicting nature, may constitute the "stress" component. It is relatively easy to imagine how the alteration of neurotransmitter activity alters connectivity in the brain; however, it is much more difficult to imagine how external stimuli (e.g., stressful life events) interfere.

An analogy of "conflict" may explain the disruptive influences that external stressful stimuli may have on the connectivity of the brain. Environmental external information has a constraining influence on the networks that process incoming information. Imagine that two or more external inputs constrain a network to assume opposing configurations. Units of the network will tend to assume values relevant to one configuration and at the same time these units will also be constrained to assume the values of the other configuration. Since the two configurations are different, the constraints for each configuration will be different. Those units induced to satisfy constraints of one input will inevitably fail to satisfy the constraints of the other. The result is a violation of constraint satisfaction that leads to connectivity breakdown in the network.

Naturally, conflicts are typically resolved one way or the other in the sense that the network converges to satisfy only one set of constraints. In effect, this is presumably the underlying mechanism of arriving at a mental solution (Rumelhart and McClelland 1986; Herz *et al.* 1991). However, imagine that the conflict is "strong," in which case the environmental message has either multiple conflicting aspects, or that the conflicting aspects strongly constrain the connectivity. Such conditions have a threatening potential to "split apart" or "fragment" the pattern of connectivity. Extensive violations of multiple constraint satisfaction could occur and destroy the functional connectivity of the system. In effect, if one examines which are the salient characteristics of environmental stresses, it seems they involve multiple strong alterations in the environment (e.g., natural disasters or wars), or a few single yet highly significant life events (e.g., death of a spouse or loved one). Such changes introduce "abrupt" new constraints to the networks of information processing and may result in rapid violation of old constraints, thereby endangering the integrity of the connectivity dynamics.

From the developmental point of view, experience-dependent plasticity is important for the organization of the brain. If an individual is reared in an environment that is characterized by inconsistency and confusion, his or her brain organization will inevitably be influenced. Continuous conflicting messages during development could damage the development of connectivity within relevant neural systems.

A substantial body of research from the 1970s concerning families of schizophrenia patients (Leff 1987; Sadock and Sadock 2004) supports this developmental concept. The idea of "double bind" proposed by Betson indicates conflicting messages at the communication level of the "schizophrenogenic family" (Gross *et al.* 1954). Wayne coined the term "pseudomutuality" to describe the finding of communication deviances in families of schizophrenia patients (Ariety and Goldstein 1959). In general, there is substantial evidence that schizophrenia patients have developmental disturbances (Weinberger 1987) to the extent that as of recently, a prodrome that predicts psychosis is being formulated (Klosterkotter 1992).

As previously noted, the systems approach to brain organization may also provide for a developmental model that explains why schizophrenia emerges between the ages of 18 and 25. Consider an interactive process of organizational function between the brain system and the environment system. Let us assume that an organizational parameter and an organizational influence are relevant to the interaction between the developing brain and the environmental organization. An infant brain is not organized and is developing to higher levels of organization partly by experience-dependent plasticity, or the organizational capacity imposed on him or her by the environment, which in this case is the family system. The organizing influences are embodied within parental upbringing and education. One may assume that at this stage the organizational influences from the environment to the infant brain are predominant, while infant organizational influences on the environment are practically zero.

As the infant matures to adulthood, the direction of predominant organizational influence is reversed. Leaving the comfort of a supportive family environment, the individual is left at the mercy of an unorganized and unfamiliar environment. Since the adult brain has acquired the organizational capacity to influence his or her environment, the adult organizes his or her environment by initiating a family of his or her own. The adult strives to order his or her environment with a constant lifestyle of daily routine. Thus, the interaction of the adult with his or her environment is characterized by a "vector" of organizational influence directed to the environment as opposed to the infant, which can only receive organizational influence from the environment.

This dynamic interaction of organizational influences reveals why early adulthood is such a vulnerable period in brain development. Early adulthood is the time when the person leaves the comfort and support of home for an unordered, independent, unfamiliar life. The young adult may have not yet achieved any organizing effect on his or her environment. During this period both brain and environmental organizations are at their lowest levels. Having barely achieved adult brain organization and having to deal with the disordered environmental challenges put the individual in a low threshold level of organization in both his or her personal and environmental systems. During this phase, organizational influences are balanced. The vector of organizational power from the brain system toward the environment system is balanced by the inverse influences from the environmental system toward the brain system. It is a critical phase transition that will eventually determine if the person will achieve the level of brain organization which will enable that individual to organize his or her life as a mature adult.

If for some reason the brain system does not achieve the threshold organization level to make the phase transition, it will result in a collapse of organization levels due to the overwhelming disorganization influences of the environmental system. This threshold dynamic of phase transition may explain the multiple factors that are considered to cause schizophrenia, such as the "stress diathesis" model. If some developmental impairment, including haphazard upbringing due to a malfunctioning family, impairs brain organizational development, then the threshold for organization capacity will not be achieved. On the other hand, normal development but an overly irregular environment that acts to disorganize the brain will also impair the threshold.

These bidirectional interactive organizational influences between environment and brain organization exemplify etiological theories of schizophrenia such as the "stress diathesis" model. Such novel explanations may bring our theories closer to brain functions. The concept of matching complexity (see previous chapters) may one day provide a mathematical formulation for putative quantitative measurements of brain–environmental interdependencies and influences. These types of theories are also in agreement with the biopsychosocial medical schools of thought.

Mood and anxiety disorders

In the previous sections depression was assumed to emerge as a property that accompanies deoptimization of internal representations. This hypothesis could be extended to assume that elevated mood accompanies optimization dynamics while depressed mood is correlated to deoptimization dynamics.

In general, three conditions can perturb the regular balance of optimization dynamics: (1) alterations in the neural substrate, (2) influences of environmental inputs such as various stressors, and (3) internal configurations "shaped by" experience-dependent processes. As already mentioned, it is known that certain "organic" factors may cause depressed mood.

The three conditions cannot be separated and once deoptimization dynamics arises, even if caused by one condition, all three conditions become implicated, making depression a sustained, prolonged, recurrent phenomenon.

Let us begin with the first condition of an altered neuronal substrate. We have already seen in previous sections that neural resilience is probably crucial to overcome a depressed mood. Neural resilience is related to depression via antidepressant medication that acts to increase neural resilience via activation of the second-neurotransmitter cascade and releases of gene activity (via activation of promoter genes) that code protein formation to increase dendrite arborization and synaptic spine formation. Increased neural resilience increases neural network flexibility and thus its adaptability to more complex and demanding computations. This flexibility allows for better optimization dynamics thus reducing deoptimization dynamics resolving depression (as the emergent property) and allowing for better mood sensations to emerge.

If increased neural resilience resolves the dynamic restriction from which depressed mood emerges, then reduction of neuronal resilience, for whatever reason, would predispose the neural network organization to deoptimization dynamics and with it to the occurrence of depression.

Neural resilience can be reduced when the input–output relations of neural activity are impaired and the transfer capabilities of dendrites to axonic connectivity are hampered. For this to occur, any neural mechanism of threshold function or synaptic transfer can be involved.

For example, hormones such as thyroid and growth factor hormones have also been found to be implicated in neuronal activity, and many hormones have recently been reclassified as neurohormones (Hokfelt *et al.* 2003). Their activity is presumably related to the activation of the G protein implemented in the second-neurotransmitter cascade activity within the cytoplasm of neural cells making up the neural network spread in the brain. Altered hormonal activity probably perturbs optimal neural reliance, reducing it and causing the neural ensembles spread in the brain to become less adaptable and less effective in the neural computation tasks demanded from them. Thus it is conceivable that hypothyroidism is likely to be accompanied by depressed mood and even full-blown clinical depression. The relationship of thyroid hormone and neural resilience probably requires in-depth research and investigation, though at this stage the relationship is putatively related to neural resilience as hyperthyroidism seems to increase neural resilience, abruptly shifting the neural network dynamics to optimization shifts which can explain why hyperthyroidism frequently accompanies manic mood swings.

If we consider the second factor that can trigger depression (i.e., the influences of environmental inputs such as various stressors), we have noted that stress has been found to reduce hippocampus volumes in animal models and that there is evidence that stress causes neural atrophy and death. This cell death and atrophy can be a direct depression-generating factor via the reduction of neural resilience that obviously accompanies neural atrophy; especially if it occurs in brain connectivity systems such as the hippocampus (connectivity systems infect global brain trajectory dynamics).

But how can we explain the fact that stressors cause neural atrophy? What is the reason that stressors, which are events and occurrences of the outside world, would have an effect on the physical construct of the neuron? Let us use our insights from neural network models and the intuitions developed so far to investigate this point.

Let us choose the death of a loved one as the stressor in discussion. Assuming we had daily interactions with the loved one, the daily interactions take the form of daily input, activating daily neural patterns related to the representation of this loved person. The loved one's death is accompanied by a cessation of the regular inputs perceived daily before his or her death, and is also a cessation of the activation of neuronal patterns that represented our daily interactions. Thus a massive neural network and numerous neural activations that were regularly activated cease. A portion of internal brain activation that used to be optimized is now dynamically deoptimized. In addition, the cessation of neural activation can directly cause the non-active neurons to die or atrophy.

This cell atrophy further increases deoptimization dynamics. From this example we may deduce that deoptimization dynamics can be triggered by stressors and subsequently maintained by consequences of the stressor (i.e., cell atrophy).

As for the last factor involved in depression, the so-called "topological internal configuration," this is linked to the loss of neuronal activation with loss of significant experience, and may be described using the same example of losing a loved one as a stressor. The internal configuration, as explained in previous sections, is the result of shaping the brain space through experience-dependent plasticity. As such, attractor formations embed internal representations of the world and relevant others. Internal configurations of attractor formations are optimized in everyday occurrences, and if there is correlation between the external occurrences and their internal representations, then optimization dynamics is balanced and eotimic (neutral) mood is the emergent property.

However, if a loved one dies, the attractor system which represents him or her in the brain system is left unmatched by the external occurrence that he or she had maintained. This mismatch is a cause for deoptimization dynamics related to that part of the brain system. Every time the loved person is remembered, the fact that he or she no longer exists shifts the system to deoptimization dynamics, explaining why such an event is typically accompanied by sadness and depressed mood.

If we examine the psychological components of stressors it is evident that loss (person or function) is one component; however, other components are typical; for example, a major life event (divorce, migration, and so on). These changes comply with the description of marked mismatch between the internal configuration (before the change occurred) and the external occurrences after the stressful change occurred. This mismatch is the trigger of deoptimization and even further cell death.

The relations of mismatch between "deviated" internal representations typical of personality disorders and the external occurrences have already been described. We can now conclude that due to the mismatch in personality disorders (caused by deviations of internal representations because of experience-dependent plasticity) even regular external occurrences can become stressors for the personality disordered patient. In this case the discrepancy between the internal representation and the external occurrence is due to the deviated internal representation (not the external occurrence) but in general the result is the same, namely a mismatch between internal and external occurrences, turning the external occurrence into a stressor just because it is not up to "internal expectations" (i.e., representations).

Thus, elderly persons are typically more exposed to depression, as their brain systems may have reduced flexibility and adaptability due to natural reductions of neural resilience (from age-related cell death or hormonal metabolic system diseases).

Three deoptimizing factors combine in the etiology of depression (i.e., organic biological, environment stressors, or personality configurations). Individually, or in combinations, these factors may trigger the deoptimization shift responsible for a clinical picture of depression. Once triggered, an "attempt" to compensate the deoptimization shift may occur, and may push the system into an oscillatory dynamic of optimizations and deoptimizations. In this case, bipolar disorder may emerge.

The law of instability states that a system subject to oscillations among a few conflicting forces is at risk of rupture and breakdown. In effect, both depression and manic disorders could develop psychosis (psychotic depression and psychosis of mania), indicating that the optimization dynamics perturbed the system enough to cause connectivity breakdown and fragmentation of the dominant brain states.

However, before connectivity is disturbed, constraint among distributed networks acts to "absorb" the agitation spread in the system. In the previous sections, anxiety was presumed to emerge from distributed frustration of constraints that accompany any disturbance of neural network organizations within the dynamics of dominant brain state. For example, destabilization of the higher level transmodal brain systems relevant to conscious awareness could be reflected by the sensation of losing control, which is typical of anxiety disorders.

In an attempt to "absorb" instabilities the perturbations typically disseminate to the rest of the nervous system including the peripheral nervous system, creating instabilities in the activities of cardiac, gastric, and other peripheral systems. Such instabilities are responsible for the somatic symptoms of anxiety (e.g., palpitations, diarrhea, and other symptoms). Thus, the variability of symptomatic manifestation of anxiety is probably correlated with the extent and distribution of destabilization within the nervous system.

As for the causes of depression, the destabilization of constraint frustration in the neural networks of the brain which emerges as anxious mood (i.e., emergent property) could arise from metabolic and toxic agents acting directly on the neural substrate, or could evolve from conflicting psychosocial events which mismatch internal configurations. Thus, anxiety has been tied to "organic" factors such as hormonal metabolic and toxic influences, as well as to personality traits and environmental stressors (Sadock and Sadock 2004).

Interestingly, most psychiatric disorders involve anxiety as a common accompanying symptom. Assuming that both optimization dynamics (i.e., mood disorders) as well as fragmentation of the dynamic dominant brain states trajectory (i.e., psychosis) are accompanied by frustration of constraints, it is plausible that anxiety is typically an accompanying symptom of most psychiatric disorders.

The idea of conflict as a reason for constraint frustration has already been addressed. If an occurrence, or event, that activates a set of brain states contradicts an internal representation or internal scheme activating an opposing organization of brain states simultaneously, then constraints between the opposing activated brain states cannot be satisfied.

The internal configuration of personality disordered patients typically mismatches the everyday occurrences of outer experiences; this actually turns the life of the personality disordered patient into a continuous conflict between "expected" internal (i.e., personal expectations) and real world events (i.e., the events in the disordered person's life). This continuous conflict is the explanation for the high level of anxiety reported by (and anxious attitudes found in) patients with personality disorders.

In the case of phobias it seems that certain situations or things can trigger destabilizations that spread out in the form of constraint frustrations among connectivity networks in transmodal brain systems. Destabilization dynamics probably follow some association patterns, as in learning. An event that was associated with destabilization of the system (or that caused by destabilization) may in some way trigger destabilization when repeated. For example, a panic attack occurring in a crowded place will create the fear and expectation that another attack will take place in a similar situation, and consequently an additional panic attack takes place, reinforcing the so-called "learned" destabilization.

Thus, while generalized anxiety is the emergent property of an unstable system characterized by frustration of constraint satisfaction, phobias and certain panic reactions are emergent properties from a stimulus-bound instability with similar frustration of constraint satisfaction.

Brain profiling

From the above descriptions, brain-related terminology that translates clusters of signs and symptoms to brain organizational disturbances can be developed. We shall call this process of relating clinical findings to brain disturbances "brain profiling." Brain profiling attempts to bridge the currently descriptive (non-etiological) diagnostic system of psychiatry with innovative brain-related psychiatric diagnoses. Figure 5.1 schematizes these relations; on the left-hand side of the figure the major signs and symptoms common in mental

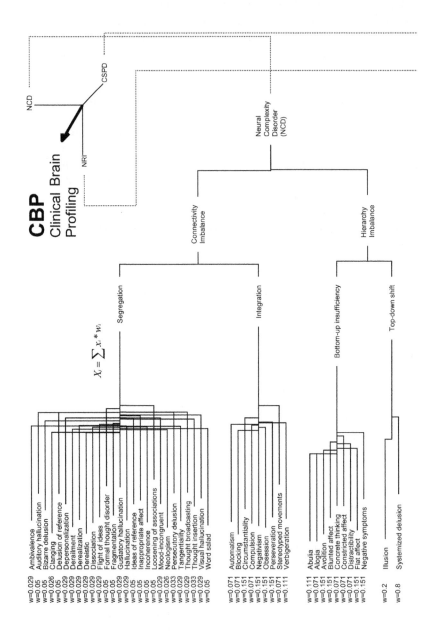

CBP
Clinical Brain
Profiling

NCD

CSPD

NRI

$$X_i = \sum x_i * w_i$$

Neural
Complexity
Disorder
(NCD)

Connectivity
Imbalance

Hierarchy
Imbalance

Segregation

Integration

Bottom-up insufficiency

Top-down shift

w=0.029	Ambivalence
w=0.05	Auditory hallucination
w=0.05	Bizarre delusion
w=0.026	Clanging
w=0.05	Delusion of reference
w=0.029	Depersonalization
w=0.029	Derailment
w=0.029	Derealization
w=0.029	Derelistic
w=0.029	Dissociation
w=0.029	Flight of ideas
w=0.029	Formal thought disorder
w=0.05	Fragmentation
w=0.029	Gustatory hallucination
w=0.029	Hallucination
w=0.05	Ideas of reference
w=0.05	Inappropriate affect
w=0.05	Incoherence
w=0.05	Loosening of associations
w=0.029	Mood-incongruent
w=0.026	Neologism
w=0.033	Persecutory delusion
w=0.029	Tangentiality
w=0.029	Thought broadcasting
w=0.029	Thought insertion
w=0.033	Visual hallucination
w=0.05	Word salad

w=0.071	Automatism
w=0.071	Blocking
w=0.151	Circumstantiality
w=0.071	Compulsion
w=0.151	Negativism
w=0.151	Obsession
w=0.151	Perseveration
w=0.071	Stereotyped movements
w=0.111	Verbigeration

w=0.111	Abulia
w=0.071	Alogia
w=0.151	Avolition
w=0.151	Blunted affect
w=0.071	Concrete thinking
w=0.071	Constricted affect
w=0.071	Distractibility
w=0.151	Flat affect
w=0.151	Negative symptoms

w=0.2	Illusion
w=0.8	Systemized delusion

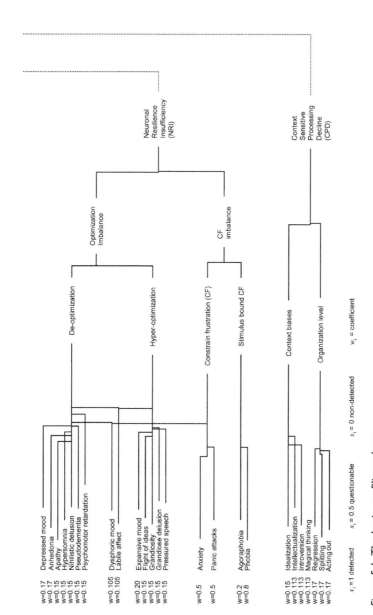

Figure 5.1 The brain profiling schema.

disorders are listed, and the hypothesized symptom-related brain disturbances clustered to a three-dimensional level of brain disturbances are listed on the right.

The brain profiling schema is designed to help the clinician quantify his or her findings by applying a weighted value "w" to each clinical finding normalizing the hypothesized brain disturbance in a three-dimensional space of brain organization. Each patient can be diagnosed for disturbances of (1) neural complexity disorders (NCD), (2) neuronal resilience insufficiency (NRI), and (3) context sensitivity processing decline (CSD) (upper right-hand part of Figure 5.1).

Neural complexity relates to the balance of connectivity and hierarchical organizations of the dominant brain states and trajectories. Brain organization may be defined as hierarchical connectivity processes going from unimodal partial segregated processes up to transmodal global integrated high-level processes. For this to take place effectively, connectivity among brain systems and units should be flexibly balanced between disconnection and over-connection dynamics. As such we are dealing with fast millisecond range processes of electrical membrane potential occurrences that continually balance the system at optimal connectivity and hierarchical dynamics.

It is obvious that connectivity balance and hierarchal balance are inseparable, and if one is disturbed the other will also suffer perturbation. Since this matrix of brain organization is balanced in the millisecond range dynamics and the changes in connectivity which accompany brain computation occur in the millisecond range, and since changes in connectivity typically assume the term of "plasticity," we may call these millisecond range alterations during brain computations "fast plasticity."

As already detailed in previous sections, brain computations of the millisecond range are related to the experience of consciousness, an experience which in itself is felt in the seconds and minutes range. We are aware of our life occurrences and ideas in a minute-by-minute time scale. Within that awareness we experience complex computations such as remembering, detecting, recognizing, and associating ideas and events under logic constraints. We use these functions in decision-making, adapting and optimizing our environment and self-expressions with others and the environment. If, for some reason, these delicate connectivity balances are perturbed and disturbed, these functions may suffer the consequences.

Conscious awareness will suffer problems of detecting, recognizing, and associating ideas and events under logic constraints. This will lead to false ideas, biased interpretations, and erroneous conclusions about the real world environment. Thus one can conclude that a news broadcast from the television is a command message from outer space to be acted upon (i.e., delusion of reference). It is thus conceivable that false ideas, delusions, loosening of associations, and biased logical reasoning will inevitably disrupt effective decision-making, adaptation, and optimization of interactions with the environment, ultimately causing the deterioration seen in individuals with schizophrenia who have suffered such maladies.

In our novel diagnosis, entities such as those of schizophrenia spectrum disorders are concordant with the idea of "neural complexity disorder" (NCD) where connectivity balances are disturbed, causing the above disturbances.

Dividing NCD into "connectivity imbalance" and "hierarchical imbalance" is artificial, as we have seen that they are interchangeable and essentially the same processes. Nevertheless, since connectivity imbalance can be more relevant to certain clinical descriptions while hierarchical imbalance is more relevant to other clinical manifestations, this division may be worthwhile.

Connectivity balance involves a balance between disconnectivity and over-connectivity; thus a disturbance to connectivity balance can take the form of "segregation" where the brain units become segregated or independent and disconnected. Alternatively, it can take the opposite form of "integrated" and become overly connected and interdependent. A disturbance of the first form (i.e., segregation) will cause the system to become unstable and random like the position of molecules in gas, while a disturbance of the second form (i.e., integration) will cause the system to become constrained and fixed, similar to the position of molecules in crystal.

In the first type of disturbances to connectivity balance (i.e., segregation) awareness will be fragmented, logic disturbed, associations loosened and altered, conclusions biased, and experience dissociated. These perturbations will be expressed as sets of symptoms and signs including delusions, loosening of associations, and ambivalence. Dissociation of multimode integration will result in hallucinations, feelings will be detached from reason with incongruent affects, and other additional disturbances of this sort will emerge. Figure 5.1 (top list on the left) details those signs and symptoms from psychiatric literature that putatively reflect segregation disturbances to the brain.

In the second type of disturbances to connectivity balance (i.e., integration), the flexibility of the brain organization will be reduced, and the tendency of processes to constrain each other will drive the brain to repeatedly constrained states; thus ideas will repeat themselves, causing perseverative obsessive and ruminant ideation. The reduced flexibility will "fixate" the brain system, reducing the number of states it can assume, and brain space will actually be reduced (see space-state formulations in previous chapters) along with ideation and experience. Poverty of speech will result from reduction of activated brain states, and the individual's total adaptability and interest in the external world will be reduced or even abolished. This is typical of the deficit negative symptoms described in schizophrenia.

Connectivity balance is therefore directly related to hierarchical balance. If integration occurs, it also constrains and damages the hierarchical organization. If connectivity is disturbed, higher level organization that depends on increased connectivity dynamics cannot be achieved. This risks a collapse of higher level transmodal formations in the brain. In effect it is most probable that in deficit syndromes (such as those of residual schizophrenia) higher level formations are insufficient. As already mentioned, this is most evident in the finding of hypo-frontality where pre-frontal lobe activity is insufficient and coupled by disturbances to high-level working memory capabilities. Thus it is possible that connectivity imbalance toward integration will also alter hierarchical balance toward "bottom-up insufficiency" (see Figure 5.1). Complicated phenomena such as "volition" probably appear as emergent properties from higher level organizations, and if these become insufficient the consequences of "abulia" described for residual schizophrenia patients and some frontal lobe patients can be explained.

Hierarchical imbalance does not involve only bottom-up processes that occur in "bottom-up insufficiency"; it can also be disturbed downward where prevailing top-down processes cause hierarchical balance to cause a "top-down shift." In this case information represented in higher level organization such as context and schemata becomes very dominant, risking the bias of incoming "upward traveling" evidence and information that forms the environment of the real world. The mismatch between the occurrences of the outer world and their representations in the contextual inner experience will take the form of a bias, and events will be experienced with a bias toward their internal higher level representations. If, for example, a contextual schema involves ideas about intrigues that should arouse suspicion, new experiences will be interpreted as menacing and threatening even if they are random or of unrelated themes. This top-down bias will cause information to be incorporated in a biased manner, gradually building up the biased schema or context to the extent that with time it is removed from reality and thus delusional. These types of delusion build up gradually starting as biases of real events. They are not bizarre and are systematic, and grow gradually but stably. In the clinical experience these are the systemized delusions attributed to delusional disorders.

As neural complexity results from fast millisecond interactions and balances, neural resilience relates to the capability of the neurons to gradually adjust to their functional role. This is achieved by processes of dendrite arboring and spine formations in the neuron. Since these processes are plasticity progressions that take days and weeks to develop, this type of plasticity may be called "slow plasticity."

Neural resilience relates to the input–output relations of each brain unit, and thus to the adaptability of constraints among brain units and states. It is conceivable that neural networks rich in dendrite arboring and spine formations turn the neural network as a whole into a much more flexible and adaptable system.

During activation and computations the space of the brain is being continually shaped and reshaped. This continuous flux of change is dependent and related to the information represented and manipulated within the brain system. If neural resilience is good, then the network made up from these resilient units is a more flexible and adaptable system resulting in more efficient neural computation capabilities. A flexible system allows computations to optimize network activity. Optimization is when the system is functioning at states that are most favorable for the computation at hand. If the conditions are too static, the more changeable configuration will be chosen and vice versa; if the condition is too changeable, the more rigid dynamics will be favored. This kind of favorable condition may be called "optimization balance," and when disturbed it becomes "optimization imbalance." Disturbances to the optimization dynamics can go either way: toward deoptimization when the system becomes less optimized, and toward hyperoptimization when the system assumes more optimized dynamics.

Since we assume that optimization dynamics is associated with mood tone as its emergent property, then we assume that deoptimizations result in suppressed mood and optimization dynamics is associated with elevated mood. During regular information processing and computations, the brain continually and simultaneously optimizes and epitomizes; thus mood shifts are minor and contra balanced, and a euthymic (i.e., stable) state generally prevails.

Deoptimization dynamics will ensue when there is a discrepancy between internal representations of attractor formation and the incoming environmental events that typically optimize them. This mismatch causes a lack of neural network activations. Instead of optimizing the attractor formations by activating matching brain states these states are not activated and as a consequence the general dynamics of the systems activity moves toward deoptimization. The mismatch can occur either because the internal configuration landscape of representations has been altered (as in altered neural resilience due to organic tissue alterations) or because the environmental input patterns change radically, as in stressful events. This explains why both internal as well as external events play a role in depression and mood alterations.

Optimization is a balanced force; thus, when depression ensues due to deoptimization dynamics, it is assumed that optimization dynamics would be triggered as a counterbalance. The optimization shift results (as an emergent property) in elevated mood. When this shift is strong and hyperoptimizes the system, manic episodes emerge. It is common to find manic episodes after depressive periods; and manic periods triggered by antidepressive medication.

Along the lines of our hypothesis of neural resilience, medication increases neural resilience by enhancing spine formation and dendrite arborization. This in turn generates more flexibility in the networks involved which then rapidly allow optimization of computations, enabling an optimization shift. Once triggered, if this dynamic optimization becomes hyperoptimized a manic episode results.

As shown in Figure 5.1, deoptimization and hyperoptimization are disturbances of optimization balance (i.e., optimization imbalance in Figure 5.1). If the system starts to oscillate between these two dynamics a clinical description of bipolar disorder appears as the emergent property. The homeostatic mechanism of biological systems can be the driving force for such oscillating dynamics as the tendency to counterbalance sets off the oscillations.

The various perturbations spread within the neural network systems during these dynamic changes and cause frustration of constraint (i.e., constraints are not satisfied; see previous chapters). Thus, in addition to the optimization imbalance constraint frustration (CF) imbalance can occur, with anxious mood as an emergent property. This can be stimulus bound, triggered by an external event, or can remain general and unrelated to any event. The former condition is typical to phobias while the latter is described as generalized anxiety disorder.

Context-sensitive processing decline (CPD) is a general term for alterations in internal representations (i.e., context), resulting in a decline in context-related processes.

There are two potential aberrations for context that can occur independently or simultaneously; first, context can be biased in relation to the external world of psychosocial events and occurrences, and second, it can be immature, having remained at lower organization levels (see previous chapters). It is clear that if context is undeveloped it will also be biased and will mismatch external events; thus undeveloped immature context formations are a more severe type of CPD. Complex observations rather than symptoms are indicators for CPD.

Magical thinking, a mode of experience of young toddlers, regression, splitting and acting out are all related to low-level personality organizations. Regression is behavior appropriate for a toddler, splitting is the type of experience when object relations did not mature, and acting out is the response of an immature system.

Intellectualization, idealization, and introversion are more related to biased modes of processing than to low-level object relations or context processing. These are only preliminary representatives indicating possible context-processing biases.

Based on previous sections it is suggested that those descriptions made by object relation theoreticians such as Kernberg and Kohut regarding severe personality disorders would be classified as CPD of lower level organization while personality disorders that have a relatively mature ego formation, and are dependent typically on alterations that result from the use of diverse defense mechanisms, will be classified as CPD of the biased type.

How does brain profiling work? First, the clinician is asked to identify the clinical manifestation in his or her patient. Scales that have spectrum coding (from 1 to 5 or 1 to 7) typically introduce "statistical noise" in the form of large subjective standard deviations. To curb this effect the identification of the clinical manifestation is limited to three coded aspects: "non-detected" coded "zero," "detected" coded "one," and questionable coded 0.5. Whenever possible it is recommended to avoid coding "questionable," especially when such coding arises from diagnostic laziness. Thus the brain profiling diagnosis requires scrutinizing interviews and in-depth clinical investigations. The detected codes (X_i) form a "diagnostic input vector" (DIV) with the number of entries equal to the number of clinical detections. When achieved, the DIV concludes the clinician's role in brain profiling diagnosis.

Not all clinical manifestations that make up the DIV have the same "strength" in indicating specific brain disturbances. Coefficients (w_i) are assigned based on the theoretical assumptions about the contribution of each detected item. Coefficients also act to normalize calculated results for different clusters. This is because clusters are not equal in the number of detected categories (for example, coding results for segregation involve twenty-seven entries, while for integration they involve only nine entries). Coefficients are subject to debate and require further clinical research. An intuitive assignment is presented (Figure 5.1, left-hand column) as a starting point. Notably, the research for determining coefficients lends well to statistical neural network models where "weighted" values may act as coefficient values.

Once the DIV is obtained and the weighted coefficients are known, assigning numerical values to the relevant brain dynamic disturbances is calculated by the relevant equation (top of Figure 5.1). The calculation progresses iteratively from lower level clustering to final three-level clustering (from left to right in Figure 5.1). Thus once obtained for segregation, integration, bottom-up insufficiency, top-down shift, deoptimization, hyperoptimization, CF, and stimulus-bound CF, it is calculated for connectivity imbalance, hierarchy imbalance, optimization imbalance, and CF imbalance. Finally, a three-dimensional estimation is calculated including neural complexity disorder (NCD), neural resilience insufficiency (NRI), and context-sensitive processing decline (CSPD).

Plotted as a three-dimensional graph (top right of Figure 5.1) or as a three-point graph in Figure 5.2 (case examples), the brain profiling method unifies in a one-point three-dimensional plot an integrative diagnosis of all relevant brain disturbances hypothesized for the diagnosed patient. Note that even though the brain profiling method culminates in a three-digit code, information is not lost and can be traced back to the full information embedded in the DIV.

One practicality of brain profiling is immediately apparent. This new diagnostic approach is a brain profiling rather than a patient stigmatizing approach. Having a malfunctioning brain is less stigmatizing than being a mentally ill person. As for coding purposes (for insurance companies and billing), the three-digit code is clinically informative, unlike the DSM codes that are not clinically related.

A much more relevant advantage of the brain profiling diagnosis is inherent in its name. It is brain oriented, offering a set of testable predictions for imaging studies of patients with relevant clinical findings. One of the shortcomings of the DSM diagnostic system according to the DSM V research agenda (Kupfer *et al.* 2005) is that the DSM-defined entities hamper research. The brain profiling diagnosis is designed to enhance research, specifically neuroimaging research that is promising *in vivo* research for mental disorders. Methods of signal analysis such as "independent component analysis" (Makeig *et al.* 1996) and "dynamic causal modeling" (Klaas *et al.* 2006) are already in a position to identify presumed brain connectivity imbalances. Diagnosing patients using brain profiling will be a turning point, and relevant imaging findings (EEG, fMRI) regarding mental disorders will become apparent.

Since brain profiling relates to synaptic plasticity, pharmacotherapy would need to be prescribed to one or more of the profiling dimensions. For example, SSRIs are relevant to neuronal resilience so they will putatively specifically address brain profiles of optimizations and constraint frustration. A more specific design of synaptic modulating medications would require brain-related diagnostic evaluation such as the brain profiling approach.

Follow-up at a glance will contribute to improved patient care in clinical settings by focusing treatment planning and clinical decision-making. The three-dimensional one-point plot of the brain profiling approach turns to a trajectory plot upon multiple assessments over time (each point in the plot is one time-related point assessment, and connecting all points creates a trajectory). The trajectory presents an easy-to-see clinical history of the patient. History plot diagrams of many patients would be valuable information to epidemiologically validate the brain profiling approach for consistency and possible entity-driven classifications. In Figure 7.1 (see Chapter 7) the three-point graphs show rough estimations using a simple computer program based on the above proposed brain profiling diagram.

Collecting clinical data

The theory of NeuroAnalysis is a conceptual outlook on mental disorders as brain disorders; however, it is also intended to pave the way for a more reliable objective diagnostic system that would be much less susceptible to biases of inter-rater reliability. However, at the present stage of development NeuroAnalysis has not produced empirical data and therefore has only theoretical potential for a futuristic objective psychiatric diagnostic system.

NeuroAnalysis is not only a theory, it is also a perspective for clinical observations. The mental tools that one uses to make clinical assessments are bound to influence these assessments. Thus Neuro-Analysis formulations and theory may have a novel influence on the way patients are diagnosed even before it has been effectively proven (or refuted).

Using the DSM diagnostic approach the clinician is conditioned to think in terms of categories and entities. DSM conceptualization involves compartmentalization of clinical findings. A weakness of this method is expressed by the conceptualization of "schizoaffective" as a disorder of "compromise" between clinical reality and the DSM categorization method. DSM initially established schizophrenia as a diagnostic entity and mood disorders such as depression as a different entity. When evaluating a patient, the clinician had to classify him or her to one of the categories, assuming (according to DSM methodology) that the patient would have one set of symptoms pertaining either to the depressive clinical manifestation or to the schizophrenia set of symptoms and signs. In reality many patients simultaneously have signs and symptoms of both schizophrenia and depression.

When using the DSM the clinician was compelled to disregard one set of symptoms if he or she wanted to make a DSM-related diagnosis. If the clinician felt that the patient was having symptoms and signs related to schizophrenia but was also depressed to a lesser degree, he or she would have to disregard the depression symptoms in order to diagnose schizophrenia. Alternatively, if depression was dominant the clinician would have to disregard the symptoms and signs of schizophrenia. It is easy to see how diagnostic information relevant to the treatment and understanding of the patient is lost using this method. Later editions of the DSM added a newer entity called schizoaffective disorder, which combines both symptomatic categories and allows for placing the patient in an "intermediate" position. This example illustrates the reality of clinical manifestation, which occurs on a spectrum, as is evident from additional DSM diagnostic entities that are periodically added.

Even more important, this example shows that the medical model of categorization of entities with specific etiologies (causes) and treatments does not adequately reflect the complexity of brain-related disturbances. The brain profiling outlook enables a spectrum evaluation as the diagnosis culminates at a point in a three-dimensional space of pathology. This in itself radically changes the outlook of the clinician and is bound to influence the clinical interview and thus the final evaluation.

It is conceivable that during the clinical interview and assessment of the patient the clinician conducts his or her questions and investigation according to a clinical model which guides his or her thought process. If the psychiatrist is guided by DSM philosophy he or she will conduct an interview that searches for categories of symptoms and so forth. This is radically different from a diagnostic interview by a psychologist who may be looking for defense mechanisms, drives, and object reorientations. Thus the theoretical framework which the clinician uses for clinical investigation seems to be of great importance and relevance to the clinical findings in the evaluation and diagnosis.

Both the psychological diagnosis and the DSM diagnosis were found to be beneficial to a certain extent; however, both are incomplete, each due to its specific limitations. The DSM is restricted to categorized signs and symptoms, and is thus less concerned with developmental and psychological dynamic interchanges, which at times may not even be considered. Psychological formulations emphasize dynamic processes and do not call attention to specific stable clinical manifestations.

Clinical brain profiling (CBP) attempts to expand the diagnostic spectrum by considering both of these extreme approaches. As such, CBP is also an attempt to influence the outlook of the clinician during the assessments of patients. The benefits of CBP include: (1) a flexible system approach, and dimensional spectrum by nature; (2) reconciliation of psychological and biological formulations under the joint framework of computational neuroscience and systems theory, and (3) clinician awareness of diagnosing complex brain perturbations and disturbances that must consider brain organization (and disorganization) when diagnosing mental disorders.

It has long been recognized that the observation itself modifies the observed phenomena (the act of putting a thermometer in water to measure its temperature alters the water temperature). Brain disturbances do not change due to clinical evaluation of the patient, but the research and clinical questions raised by the novel CBP approach may open up new possibilities and horizons for understanding and investigating mental disorders.

In general, the clinician using CBP for patient assessment should first envision the patient's brain as a complex dynamic system (composed of interacting units), that is as balanced and stable as it is dynamic and flexible. The balanced stability is robust to certain degrees but small collective changes, as well as big solitary alterations, can tip-off the balance of the system, creating massive dynamic changes to the system. These changes may be gradual or drastic phase transitions. The system can be envisioned as a flowing river with repeatedly stable patterns of currents. The units are the water molecules, and the currents and waves are their integrated interactivity outcome. The system may also resemble a large orchestra, where the musicians are the units and their integrated interactive activity is expressed as music (the music being the emergent property of the orchestra's activity as a whole).

However, the recommended approach for the clinician using CBP is to imagine the occurrences in the brain of the patient being evaluated. The advantage of visioning the brain itself as the dynamic system lies in the need to have firsthand excellent knowledge of neuroanatomy neuroscience, neural computation, and neural-network sciences, all these conceptualized in the framework of dynamic systems behaviors. This recommendation actually defines the scientific curriculum that the psychiatrist of the future will have to master in addition to the one currently applied in medical training of psychiatry.

There is currently no objective brain-related diagnosis for mental disorders, but hopefully implementation of CBP will encourage physicians to ask direct brain-related clinical questions that would be investigated according to the testable prediction approach that the CBP would generate. The findings from such research would develop the CBP model, and thus in an interactive manner of clinical evaluations and clinical research a definitive brain-related diagnostic system will ultimately be developed for psychiatry.

The clinician should thus be aware of the importance of developing appropriate clinical skills and experience to extract the most accurate and irrefutable clinical evaluation based on concise in-depth accurate investigations of signs and symptoms.

A useful diagram that the clinician can use in translating clinical findings to neural system theory is presented in Figure 5.2. In this figure squares represent the hypothesized brain dynamics and circles represent observable clinical findings and anamnesis data collections. Thus translation progresses from circles to squares.

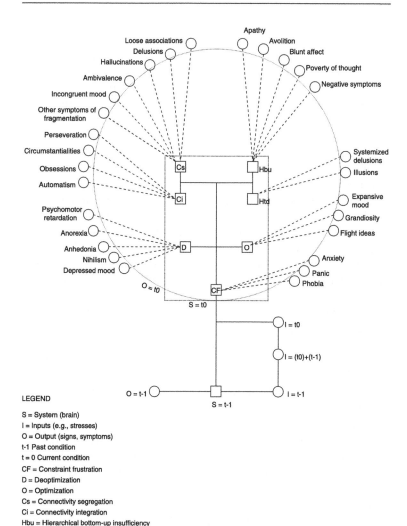

Figure 5.2 Brain profiling.

The system approach of brain organization follows two main ideas: the idea of input-system-output dynamics and the idea of different patterns of disturbed brain system organization. Thus, in Figure 5.2, "S" stands for system, accordingly "I" stands for input and "O" for output. The system (the brain system) has a history, a developmental past, and thus is represented by the mathematical symbol of "t-1"; thus S = t-1 is the condition of the system in the past. I = t-1 and O = t-1 are the input and output of the system in the past. These are represented as circles, meaning that the clinician has to gain information about the conditions of the brain system in the past via its past inputs and outputs. In other words, the clinician needs to know the past conditions within which the system developed.

The inputs (I = t-1) are the experiences, stressors, stimuli, and occurrences that characterized the patient in the past from infancy to adulthood. The outputs (O = t-1) are assessments of the patient's behaviors, complaints, signs, and symptoms in the past from infancy to adulthood. Is there information about behavioral problems, problems of adaptation, specific complaints, and disturbances?

Both past inputs I = t-1 and outputs O = t-1 give an idea of the development of the system S = t-1. Did it evolve optimally? Did it suffer perturbations or instabilities, leaving it vulnerable and thus less effective for computations in adulthood?

S = t0 (large square in Figure 5.2) is the definition of the system at time zero, meaning at the moment of evaluation. Input at the time of evaluation (I = t0) provides information about any stressor or condition that is relevant to the organization of the system either perturbing the organization causing disturbances, or enhancing organization protecting it from perturbation. The output O = t0 represents the observations of the system in terms of behaviors, signs, and symptoms.

It is important to gain information about current stressors that in combination with past experience (past relevant stressors) can cause special disturbing effects to the system. This information needs to be collected by the clinician and as such is represented by a circle coded I = (t0) + (t-1).

As already mentioned, the output O = t0 represents the observations of the system in terms of behaviors, signs, and symptoms. Major relevant clinical findings are presented as circles "positioned around" the current brain system organization (the circle around the big square of S = t0). Each circle with its relevant clinical finding points to a specific square within S = t0, and these squares are indicators of the hypothesized brain disturbance. The presumed brain disturbances are hierarchically schematized from the bottom up. CF stands for constraint frustrations and is a minor perturbation respective to optimization imbalance (D standing for deoptimization shifts and O for optimization shifts: Figure 5.2). Perturbations to the connectivity balances are more severe than those to optimization dynamics and constraints.

As such, this hierarchy represents patterns of clinical manifest-ations; the perturbation with higher, more severe consequences also involves those of lower levels but not conversely, the disturbances for lower levels do not necessarily involve higher level disturbances. Clinically this is evident, as psychotic patients also suffer from symp-toms of mood and anxiety disturbances while patients of pure anx-iety disorders do not necessarily also have mood and psychotic symptoms.

Figure 5.2 offers the clinician a framework that integrates his clini-cal findings, translating them into brain system conceptualization. At the end of the evaluation, according to the schema of Figure 5.2, the clinician can begin to formulate a proposed hypothesis of brain disturbances for his patient. He can see if the brain organization is hampered by past occurrences and developmental flaws, or if, in addition, a relevant stressor further perturbed the system. He can evaluate the severity of the disturbance. Is it a mainly low level of perturbation to constraint organization or is it severe to the extent of disturbing connectivity altogether? Effective clinical observation can further determine if connectivity is totally disrupted or partially disrupted, involving only certain subsystems of the brain.

Developing the schemata of Figure 5.2 and integrating it with Figure 5.1 can eventually provide the clinician with an effective transnational framework of mental disorders to brain disturbances, one that can serve as a comprehensive testable prediction for the underlying disturbances of mental disorders.

Chapter 6

Implications for future directions and therapy

What are the implications of the above formulations for the future, especially for the future of therapy? The approach presented may lead to the conceptualization of more effective therapeutic interventions in the future. It is evident that in order to improve brain organization, effective control over plasticity must be achieved. Improved brain organization is relevant for "corrective" interventions involving disturbances that have been consolidated. In effect it would be extremely beneficial if brain connectivity could be controlled to allow for higher plasticity dynamics. In effect this would be allowing brain plasticity to become pliable, as in the early developmental years, when it is amenable to change and reshaping. Thus a basic condition for any corrective therapeutic activity in the brain involves "synaptogenetic control." Once synaptogenesis is increased there will be a need for an additional intervention in order to create a synaptogenetic change, in accord with Hebbian dynamics (described in Chapter 3). Two categories of interventions will be necessary: "experience control" and direct "brain pacing."

As explained previously, experience "shapes" plasticity and connectivity organizations via experience-dependent plasticity; thus by controlling the experience of a patient one could control the connectivity and plasticity changes relevant for therapy. "Virtual reality" produced using modern multimedia computer technology has the potential for experience control (explained below). Another method for enhancing association between activations of neuronal ensembles is by directly activating (or inhibiting) them with electrical currents (deep brain stimulations) or magnetic inductions (transcranial magnetic stimulation (TMS)) as follows.

Synaptogenic control

Recently, the long-held view that neurogenesis in the human brain ceases after birth has been challenged. It is known today that new cells are born (i.e., stem cells) in the periventricular zones and migrate to cortical and hippocampal regions making regional and even more distanced functional cortical connections (Kukekov *et al.* 1999). This growth is increased when injury occurs and also with intensive training within stimuli-rich environments.

Certain neurohormones and growth factors generate new cells in the brain; for example, fibroblast growth factor (FGF) injected subcutaneously in rats successfully passes the blood brain barrier (BBB) and increases cell and synaptic growth (Xian and Gottlieb 2001). However, evidence suggests that in humans FGF may induce brain tumors (Berking *et al.* 2001), making this factor inappropriate for treatment.

A better candidate for inducing neurogenesis in the human brain could involve neurotransmitter agonists and antagonists. The activity of serotonin and norepinephrine has been found to participate in cell growth. Chronic antidepressant treatment has been found to increase neurogenesis of hippocampal granule cells via postreceptor increase of AMP (Thompson *et al.* 2000). Agonists of serotonin for 5HT1A and other receptors have also been mentioned as important neurogenetic factors (Lotto *et al.* 1999). In effect, serotonin depletion during synaptogenesis leads to decreased synaptic density and learning deficits in the adult rat (Mazer *et al.* 1997). Tianeptine, a 5HT1A agonist, blocks stress-induced atrophy of CA3 pyramidal neurons (Magarinos *et al.* 1999). Intrathecal treatment with quipazine (another serotonin agonist) has improved locomotion deficit induced by ventral and ventrolateral spinal neural injury (T13) in two cats. Both cats recovered quadrupedal voluntary locomotion and maintained regular steeping with this treatment (Brustein and Rossignol 1999). Sumatriptan (CPP) is a 5HT agonist (5HT2C, 5HT1D, and 5HT1A agonist) typically used in the treatment of migraine headaches, and chronic administration of sumatriptan has been found to slightly improve OCD patients (Hwang and Dun 1999).

Additional findings relevant to neurogenesis involve electroconvulsive seizures (ECS), and chronic ECS administration-induced sprouting of granule cells in the hippocampus (Kondratyev *et al.* 2001; Lamont *et al.* 2001). This effect is dependent on repeated ECS treatment and is long-lasting (observed up to at least six months after the last ECS treatment). Excitotoxin and kindling-induced sprouting are thought to be, at least in part, an adaptation in response to the death of target neurons. In contrast, there is no evidence of cell loss or dying neurons in response to chronic ECS (Gombos *et al.* 1999).

In recent years attention has been directed toward N-Methyl-D-aspartic acid (NMDA) receptor and alpha-amino-3-hydroxy-5-methyl1-4-isoxasole propionic acid (AMPA) receptors due to their apparent role of regulating neural plasticity. The L-quinoxalin-6-ylcarbonyl piperadine (CX516) AMPA modulator has the potential to control certain neuronal plasticity processes (Lynch and Gall 2006).

CX516 was tested as a sole agent in a double-blind placebo-controlled design in a small series of patients with schizophrenia (n=6) who were partially refractory to treatment with traditional neuroleptics. The study entailed weekly increments in doses of CX516, from 300mg tid for week one up to 900mg tid at week four. Patients were followed with clinical ratings, neuropsychological testing, and were monitored for adverse events. Four patients received two to four weeks of CX516, two received a placebo and two withdrew during the placebo phase. Adverse events associated with drug administration were transient and included leukopenia in one patient and elevation in liver enzymes in another. No clear improvement in psychosis or in cognition was observed over the course of the study. CX516 at the doses tested did not appear to yield dramatic effects as a sole agent, but inference from this study is limited (Marenco *et al.* 2002).

CX516 was also added to clozapine in four-week, placebo-controlled, dose-finding (N=6) and fixed-dose (N=13) trials. CX516 was tolerated well and was associated with moderate to large, between-group effect sizes compared with the placebo, representing improvement in measures of attention and memory. These preliminary results suggest that CX516 and other "ampakines" hold promise for the treatment of schizophrenia (Goff *et al.* 2001).

As mentioned above, synaptogenic interventions alone would probably have no therapeutic effect. Synaptogenic interventions would serve as promoters, enhancers, or basic requirements, for experience control and direct "brain pacers" (see below).

Experience control

Before discussing "experience-control," it must be emphasized that this type of control is presumed to have efficacy only if adjuvant effective relevant synaptogenetic medication is administered.

Experience control should include emerging computer technology of virtual reality (VR) that provides for interactive control over the senses and enables the creation of controlled environments and two-way interplay. VR is a set of computer technologies which, when combined, provide an interactive interface to a computer-generated world. Virtual reality technology (VRT) combines real-time computer graphics, body tracking devices, visual displays, and other sensory input devices to immerse a participant in a computer-generated virtual environment. He can then see, hear, and navigate in a dynamically changing scenario in which he participates as an active player modifying the environment via his interventions. This technology provides such a convincing interface that the user often believes that he or she is actually in the three-dimensional computer-generated environment. The term "presence" was coined by the experts of VRT to describe this conviction.

The field in which VRT is currently most intensively investigated in psychiatry is that of exposure therapy for treating anxiety disorders such as phobias and PTSD (Glantz and Lewis 1997; Rothbaum *et al.* 2000; Jo *et al.* 2001; Pertaub *et al.* 2001; Vincelli *et al.* 2001). In traditional exposure therapy, the subject is exposed to anxiety-producing stimuli while allowing the anxiety to attenuate with the aid of various relaxation techniques. VRT enables low-cost (flight phobia treatment without really flying), time-saving (from therapist's office) and controlled (the phobic stimulus can be designed and controlled) virtual phobic environmental exposures.

VRT has an excellent potential both for neuropsychological assessment as well as for cognitive rehabilitation. There are already a few research groups experimenting with VRT for cognitive rehabilitation (Christiansen *et al.* 1998). Traditional neuropsychological testing methods are limited to measurements of specific theoretically predetermined functions such as short-term memory or spatial orientation. Given the need to administer these tests in controlled environments, they are often highly contrived and lack ecological validity, or any direct translation to everyday functioning (Rizzo and Buckwalter 1997).

VR technology enables subjects to be immersed in complex

environments that simulate real world events and challenge mental functions more ecologically. While existing neuropsychological tests obviously measure some brain-mediated behavior related to the ability to perform in an "everyday" functional environment, VR could enable cognition to be tested in situations that are ecologically valid. While quantification of results in traditional testing is restricted to predetermined cognitive dimensions, with VR technology, many more aspects of the subjects' responses could be quantified. Information on latency, solution strategy, visual field preferences, and so on could be quantified. VR can immerse subjects in situations where complex responses are required and the responses can then be measured (Rizzo and Buckwalter 1997).

These capabilities may potentially act upon diagnosed brain deficiencies. For example, performing within virtual environments that require intensive activation of working memory would enhance the integration of higher level contextual systems. If additional multimodal integration is required to perform within that environment, then additional multimodal integration will be enhanced.

Virtual environments could also target delusional ideations and attempt to correct them by providing opposing or "correctional" occurrences tailored to counteract the specific false ideation. The correctional situations provide additional possible interpretations of the situation, thus increasing the number of possible interpretations and increasing differentiation in the representational contextual system. Performance within complex social situations that require theory-of-mind capabilities would enhance the higher level brain integration needed to represent and perform within socially cued situations.

In sum, VRT in diagnosis and rehabilitation of mental disorders could have a significant role both for increasing integration as well as differentiation by exposing the patient to complex, challenging, expressly designed interactive virtual environments.

Drawing upon the theory of experience-dependent plasticity, it is presumed that many sessions with the predesigned virtual experience will eventually "reconnect" and reassociate the neuronal network circuitry required to re-establish consistent and coherent everyday experiences for the patient. Thus, if there are no speaking figures in the immediate experience, hallucinatory voices should disappear. It is predicted that once experience control sessions are stopped and speaking figures disappear the voices will also vanish. The newly formed consistency in the system will inhibit the activation of voices without their counterparts of experience (i.e., will not enable inconsistencies of experience). The end result could be a reduction of hallucinations, providing symptomatic relief for the patient. Delusions could be treated by repeated sets of virtual experiences where delusional thinking contrasts with the virtual events. For example, a patient who is convinced of being persecuted by the FBI might be virtually introduced to the FBI headquarters where he experiences warm and caring acceptance, with no evidence of persecution. Gradually, this type of repeated "corrective experience" "improving experience?" might alter his delusion, reducing its threatening content. One may argue that delusions are unshakable beliefs and thus could never be altered. Nevertheless, clinical experience shows us that beliefs may come in various degrees from normal and overvalued ideas to real delusions. Intensive and repeated virtual experiences delivered in an "aggressive" and "focused" manner to the specific delusional system of the patient may turn delusions into overvalued ideas or even into normal thinking.

It should be noted that conventional psychotherapy is also a type of manipulation of experience (in the form of interactions with the psychotherapist); thus synaptogenetic medications hold the promise of being psychotherapy enhancers that enable psychotherapeutic changes normally achieved over years to be obtained in shorter periods (months).

Direct brain pacemaker control

"Brain pacemaker" control is a term reserved for manipulations directed to the neural tissue in the brain intended to enhance task-dependent neuronal integration and differentiation. Speculating on current technology, two main directions can be formulated: transcranial magnetic stimulation (TMS) pacemaker and electrode transplant DBS.

TMS is a technique introduced in 1985 (Barker et al. 1985) that uses the principle of inductance to activate nerve cells in the cerebral cortex (Hallett 2000). Current psychiatric research with TMS is conducted with the purpose of substituting electroconvulsive therapy (ECT) with magnetic stimulation in the treatment of mental disorders such as depression (Klein et al. 1999; Pridmore and Belmaker 1999). ECT is an established way of "resetting" brain activity, without much scientific basis, but with empirical success (Fogg-Waberski and Waberski 2000).

In a recent study, Klimesch and colleagues (2003) showed that rapid transcranial magnetic stimulation (TMS) induced task-related alpha desynchronization in human individuals and enhanced task performance. Hoffman and colleagues (2003) showed that TMS of <1Hz administered to the left temporoparietal cortex in drug-resistant hallucinating schizophrenics could significantly reduce the hallucinations. Since EEG, together with other imaging techniques, are beginning to reveal possible disturbances of brain organization, then coupling TMS with EEG offers new potential directions to start controlling brain functions directly by feedback EEG-dependent TMS delivery. A future potential "brain pacemaker" would probably involve a multiple-coil TMS device coupled with an EEG-dependent feedback mechanism, similar to a cardiac pacemaker set to act according to the ECG arrhythmias.

Deep brain stimulation (DBS) could be an additional direct method to control brain organization. It has been successful in patients with severe Parkinson's disease. Electrical stimulation of basal ganglia structures has been found to be crucially beneficial for these patients.

A combined effort of the three intervention modes—plasticity inductions, experience control, and direct pacing—harbor a promise to affect the brain radically enough to cure mental and personality disorders.

Chapter 7

Implications of NeuroAnalysis in clinical settings

Case reports

Nine case reports (David, Jacob, Benjamin, Samuel, Tim, John, Daniel, Sandra and Barbara: names are imaginary) illustrate the contribution of NeuroAnalysis to clinical practice. Each case is discussed using current conventional clinical and diagnostic evaluation, followed by insights gained from NeuroAnalysis. The contribution of these additional insights and the meaning of NeuroAnalysis for future potential therapies will be discussed. The reports are based on true cases, but all names and identifying factors are imaginary.

David

David is 25 years old and diagnosed with schizophrenia. He is in a rehabilitation department waiting to be transferred to a community-based hostel.

During previous trials in a hostel setting, David's condition tended to deteriorate, leading to aggressive behavior, where on occasion he attacked hostel personnel, causing serious injuries. At present, hostels in the surrounding neighborhoods are refusing to accept him because of his "reputation" for violent behavior.

David's current hospitalization in a secure ward was a court-ordered compulsory hospitalization following a violent outburst in which he threatened the hostel supervisor. He was later transferred to a rehabilitation department.

When admitted, David was tense, anxious, restless, had a menacing attitude, and threatened the staff after accusing them of persecuting him and wanting to harm him. He denied ever having hallucinations. His speech was pressured and he tended to jump from one topic to another; however, his speech was understandable and he was able to convey what he wanted to say. His menacing and hostile affect easily fluctuated to a childishly weeping affect.

An in-depth investigation of the occurrences that preceded his outburst revealed that it began when he argued with the hostel supervisor about the rules regarding vacations, which included obtaining permission to leave the hostel grounds and reporting his whereabouts.

During the months preceding his violent outburst, David regularly argued with the hostel staff when confronted with his misbehavior and repeatedly apologized and promised to abide by the rules, but he did not keep his promises and his agitation accelerated in subsequent arguments.

At admission to the secure unit, his suspiciousness and his thoughts of being mistreated by the hostel staff were readily interpreted as delusions of persecution and he was diagnosed with schizophrenia, confirming the diagnosis of paranoid schizophrenia that he received during previous hospitalizations.

His medical history revealed fifteen prior hospitalizations beginning at age 17. All of his hospitalizations were involuntary admissions following violent behavior. Hospitalizations ranged from a few weeks to a few months, and the last hospitalization was the longest. He was transferred to a rehabilitation department after spending six months in a closed ward.

When hospitalized, he received antipsychotic agents that quickly reduced and often eliminated his persecutory ideas and attitudes. He rapidly became coherent and cooperative. Once improved, he seemed very childish, insecure, and readily burst into tears, but was also easily irritated if his demands were not immediately satisfied. Although his agitated behavior sometimes subsided, he remained impatient, and he was preoccupied with short-term "rewards" such as permission to go outside, permission to smoke, and visitation rights.

During staff rounds he was very dull and constricted with a limited range of interests and attitudes. It was difficult to discuss with him any subject other than the issue of his discharge. No matter what subject the medical staff would want to discuss, he returned to the topic of when he would be discharged. During all patient evaluations David was tense and anxious.

His medical records showed that though he regularly took medication while hospitalized, he was convinced that he did not need it, that he was not sick, and that he was unjustly hospitalized. He considered hospitalization an unjust punishment. Once discharged he always stopped taking his medication; thus, following his last hospitalization, he received intramuscular long-acting antipsychotic medications administered monthly. However, he did not show up at the outpatient clinic for the second injection, and in effect terminated his pharmacotherapy. He inevitably returned to the streets and ended up on street drugs. The use of stimulants rapidly destabilized the remission achieved during hospitalization.

David's personal history is grim. His family's socioeconomic level was very low. His father was an alcoholic who beat his mother and ultimately disappeared, leaving his mother to raise seven children. His mother worked long hours as a cleaner, leaving the children to care for themselves. David's early childhood memories included walking barefoot and in the streets with his older brothers. He did not attend school, and when the welfare authorities intervened in an attempt to send him to a dormitory setting he would run away, back to the streets. When the authorities finally gave up, he joined the street life of drugs and crime.

David's childhood was spent in a violent atmosphere accompanied by serious deprivation. He barely learned to read and write, and did not receive any attention or support from his mother, and sorely lacked the parental love that every child needs. In the rehabilitation department the medical staff debated whether schizophrenia or personality disorder was the dominant diagnosis. The *Diagnostic and Statistical Manual for Mental Disorders* actually allows a multiaxis diagnosis where one axis can carry the diagnosis of schizophrenia and the other axis (i.e., axis two) can be the diagnosis of personality disorder.

Designation of a primary diagnosis was necessary in order to determine prognosis and treatment. It was suggested that perhaps David did not have schizophrenia and that his entire clinical picture could be attributed to his personality disorder and his use of street drugs. The argument for personality disorder was supported by the fact that he never actually revealed deterioration with typical negative signs of schizophrenia (abulia, autism, flat-affect, and total apathy), never had auditory hallucinations, and his persecutory ideations were not typical of schizophrenia. His "persecutory ideations" were in the context of arguments with the hostel staff when he was criticized for not obeying the rules, and his childish reaction reflected by his low frustration levels was part of an immature personality with delusions reflecting an attitude of "you are against me."

Despite this observation he was nevertheless diagnosed with

schizophrenia perhaps due to the treatment orientation that indicated a use of antipsychotic medication which is easier to administer than psychotherapy (relevant to the diagnosis of personality disorders), and more effective in terms of immediate therapeutic response (psychotherapy is long term and expensive).

Using NeuroAnalysis David's brain may be generally viewed as an unstable, undeveloped system. During hospitalizations, especially around admission, brain instability is predominant, while in between hospitalizations and toward discharge from hospitalization stability returns but the immature undeveloped brain is left as before. Instability around admissions is evidently due to connectivity imbalance of the segregated type (see Figure 7.1). Incoherence and loosening of associations are evident findings at hospitalizations (i.e., derailment, flight of ideas, and persecutory delusions are less prominent but sufficiently apparent). Scoring on these findings indicate that around hospitalizations David's brain suffers from a "neural complexity disorder" of "connectivity imbalance" "segregation" type (see Figure 7.1). Brain units act independently unconstrained by each other due to functional disconnections among them. Brain states representing ideas and concepts in David's brain are activated in a disconnected manner, thus jumping from one concept to a different, unrelated concept.

The segregated type of connectivity imbalance is also accompanied by frustrations of constraints (see Figure 7.1) in the involved, as well as the remaining brain systems, and when the concurring frustration of constraints increases with connectivity imbalance it accounts for the anxious mood observed at admissions.

Why did David have such instabilities in his brain, and how did they evolve and establish a pattern? To answer this question we can turn to the clear evidence that his brain suffered a developmental disturbance.

The conditions of his early childhood worked against mature development of the brain. Brain development in infancy and childhood is via experience-dependent plasticity. The environment into which a child is born is critically relevant to the organization of the brain. David was born in an environment of instability, inconsistency, and chaos, which made it difficult for the brain to achieve stable connectivity patterns. According to the Hebbian algorithm, neurons strengthen connections through a process of repeated activations. In a structured environment and stable upbringing there is a constancy characterized by repeating stimuli created by routine.

If, however, the environment is chaotic, unstructured, and without routine and repeated stimuli, ensembles of neurons cannot be repeatedly activated and effective connectivity cannot be established. The brain will then have weak connectivity patterns and a tendency toward random activations of neural ensembles.

As described in previous sections the landscape of internal attractor systems is also a sequence of connectivity dynamics. These attractor systems are the internal representations which develop and mature as we grow; they determine our experience of the outer world, shape our attitudes toward psychosocial events, and thereby form our personality.

For David the lack of constancy in his experiences and his chaotic upbringing has not only weakened the connectivity patterns among brain units and states; it has also hampered maturation of internal representations leaving him with rudimental partial internal representations; thus splitting, regression, and acting out are his modes of responding to occurrences. David's tendency to split precludes his ability to understand that others can have complex attitudes toward him. He does not realize that when the supervisor at the hostel criticized him, it was out of concern for his welfare. He experienced an all "bad" attitude, where the supervisor was alien and against him.

The childish attitudes that David revealed after medication took effect also reflect immature attitudes resulting from immature rudimental internal presentations of attractor formations. It is thus conceivable that in David's case we are confronted with a brain system that never fully developed as it was inherently exposed to instability. In addition, David's brain was exposed to the adjunctive destabilizing effects of street drugs. In such conditions even minor stressors such as arguments about his return schedule to the hostel could upset the balanced brain organization.

The activity of antipsychotic medication on brain organization is yet to be clarified. Putatively, antipsychotic agents stabilize functional connectivity as they "push" the brain to more stable, ordered associations and reduce delusions. This effect was revealed during David's hospitalization when his disorganized activity was reduced.

Antipsychotic agents may exert a limiting force on destabilization and thus have a certain "protective" effect for recurring destabilizations. However, to allow a more lasting therapeutic effect, the brain must achieve maturity and stability.

Psychotherapy is currently the most relevant treatment for such an endeavor. Therapeutic sessions act as experience-dependent processes

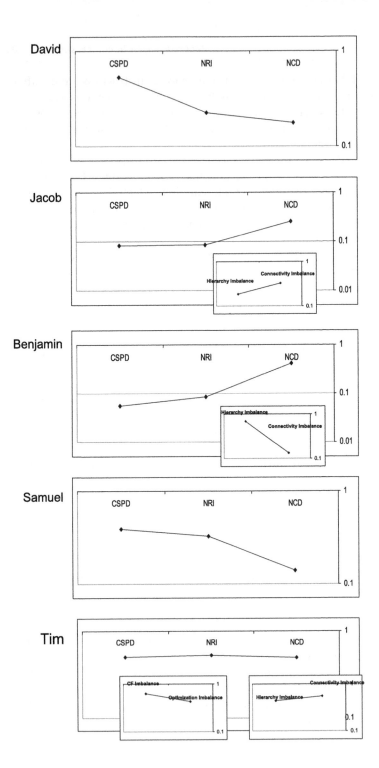

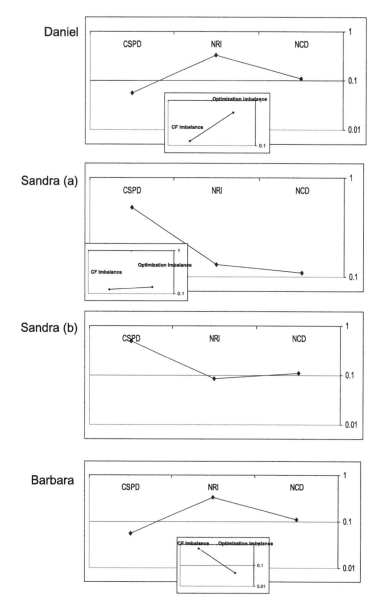

Figure 7.1 NeuroAnalysis cases.

and corrective experiences have an experience-dependent plasticity effect of increasing the complexity and efficiency of attractor systems and thus of personality maturation. Currently, this type of therapy has low efficacy, as the plasticity of the brain is reduced in adulthood and alterations necessary for an effective major change are no longer possible in adulthood.

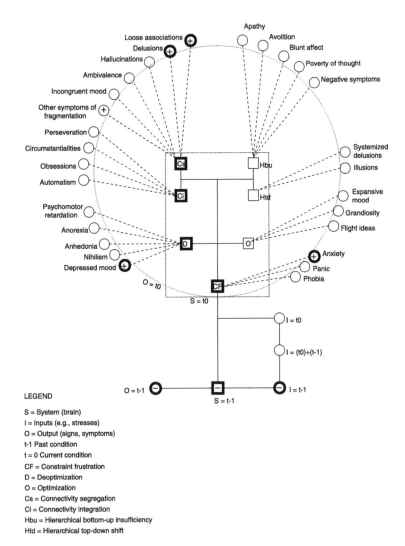

Figure 7.2 David's clinical evaluation.

Future goals for pharmacotherapy include development of plasticity-inducing medications that would allow therapists to return the treated brain to the plasticity levels of infancy, and intervene at the stage when development was hampered, to effectively remedy the deficient process. Psychotherapy would effectively contribute to more rapid results. Once brain organization and maturity is increased, the vulnerability to destabilization will be reduced, preventing the further decompensation and repeated hospitalizations.

Using the brain profiling diagnostic system, David's diagnosis can be presented by the graph in Figure 7.1. David's major problem is CSPD (context-sensitive processing decline). He also has a relatively significant impairment of NRI (neural resilience insufficiency) and NCD (neural complexity disorder) expressed by anxious moods and loosening of associations with a tendency for delusions of persecution. However, these are not his main problems and they typically reduce when he is on medication and in the supportive environment of a closed ward. CSPD, his primary disorder is not alleviated. The context-sensitive processing deficit remains in David's brain, and is the cause of repeated destabilizations and hospitalizations.

Figure 7.2 shows David's clinical evaluation on the clinician chart. The marked circles indicate findings from his clinical assessment and information from his medical history. The marked squares represent the assumed brain disturbances. The "+" sign indicates the finding at the evaluation while the "−" sign indicates findings from past hospitalizations. It is clear from Figure 7.2 that the diagnosis of David's problem is complex and involves multiple brain levels including his past development. His symptomatic profile includes psychosis, mood and anxiety symptoms, which reflect the multiple levels of his brain disturbance.

Jacob

Jacob is 45 years old and has been hospitalized for seventeen years in a semi-open department for chronic psychiatric patients. He was diagnosed with schizophrenia, paranoid type.

Jacob was born into a middle-class family, his development was normal and there were no problems with his behavior, intelligence, or cognition in his childhood. Jacob was a good student and became a computer engineer. He had a steady girlfriend and everything seemed to be going well. At age 28 he was working as a computer engineer in the navy and had a responsible job in security. He began to sense that something was wrong with his computers. One of the computers repeatedly failed and although these failures had previously occurred frequently Jacob thought that something strange was happening. He could not locate the problem, and this occupied his mind and made him anxious. Although he ultimately resolved the computer problem and repaired it as he had done many times before, he could not stop thinking about what had caused the seemingly regular failure. After a few weeks he concluded that these computer failures resulted from someone trying to penetrate his computer. When similar failures occurred in additional computers he was convinced that someone was deliberately contaminating all of the computers under his responsibility.

Although in reality his job was to repair frequently recurring computer bugs, and though nothing unusual had actually happened, he became more and more convinced that someone was penetrating his computer. As this notion gradually grew, suddenly everything took on a special meaning. Occurrences he had previously disregarded as non-relevant now became critical and confirmed his beliefs. If a cup of coffee was left on the table in an office it meant that information from the computer on that desk was stolen.

But why should anyone want to steal information? After a few days of nagging thoughts, it suddenly became clear to Jacob. It was because he was about to reveal a secret formula that would achieve ten times more energy than the atom bomb. This was valuable powerful information. He became so involved in detecting clues regarding attempts to steal his secret that he stopped functioning at work and his superiors began to ask what was going on. Jacob also received an official letter complaining about his lack of performance at work. That was when he realized that those responsible for bugging his computers were his superiors. He was convinced that they wanted to steal his secret formula. To counteract their attempted penetration of his computers he began writing letters to the supreme command of the navy about his superiors, explaining his claims and providing the clues that allegedly "proved" he was being persecuted. The response soon came, as his superiors understood that something very troublesome was happening. He was transferred to another job that did not involve computers or too much responsibility.

Now it was all clear: he had been deprived of his genius program of creating energy and by then everyone was against him. When he was alone he heard murmuring sounds of people talking behind him.

When he turned his head nobody was there but the voices did not stop.

Everything had hidden meanings: if the bus stopped near him when he was walking in the street it meant that he had to visit his brother. The world was full of conflicting meanings and thoughts jumping from one meaning to another. Associated meanings made him confused and tired. However, the thoughts running through his head made it hard for him to fall asleep and he slept for only a few hours at a time when he was totally exhausted. He was ultimately fired due to total inefficiency at his job. One day, while walking outside, he noticed a billboard with an advertisement for a tourist resort called "Solomon Islands." To Jacob it clearly meant that he was King Solomon.

During the next few days clues and meaningful events rapidly increased, the voices became stronger, and turned from unclear murmurs into repeated commands. One day an airplane flying overhead meant that he must climb up the next building, Luckily he was only on the second floor when the voices started commanding him to "jump, jump, jump." He jumped and suffered multiple fractures in both legs. At the hospital he explained that "I am King Solomon and nothing can happen to me. Even though I was taken to the hospital, in reality I am not hurt." This speech content immediately alerted the attending medical staff that a psychiatrist should be involved.

Following the psychiatric evaluation Jacob was hospitalized and diagnosed as suffering from a psychotic episode with potential to harm himself. He was put on antipsychotic medication. On the ward a fantastic content of thought was revealed; everything had a meaning, even the color of the shirt of the examining doctor. Anything that was said had a meaning and generated an association. For example, if the date had one of the letters of his name, it meant that something was going to happen, or alternatively something should happen. One day without any reason he stopped eating. Investigation revealed that when asking other patients about his age, one of the numbers correlated with the letter "f" for "food" meaning he must stop eating.

At first he was allowed to take vacations accompanied by his family, and his brother would take him home for the weekend. On one occasion his brother wore a red shirt, which Jacob associated with blood, meaning that he had to die. These associations prolonged the hospitalization, as risk was evident. Vacations ultimately had to be stopped when on one occasion he tried to attack his brother due to an association with something that was announced on the radio. He did not respond to various trials with antipsychotic agents and as time went by he was transferred to the chronic ward where he was treated with limited success. In repeated evaluations on the ward he was continuously found to have delusions of reference. Everything neutral in Jacob's environment had a special (frequently changing) meaning for him. Meanings were generated by associations. He suffered from mild to severe loosening of associations. In addition, his delusions were sometimes persecutory.

His affect was largely incongruent. He would say, for example, that his brother must die, while he was laughing and seemingly in a good mood. At times, he was occupied with terrible thoughts; however, he was only mildly anxious or not anxious at all. He constantly heard voices as was evident from his hallucinatory behavior. He would assume a listening attitude during interviews as if someone other than the examiner was talking to him. When asked, he would not conceal that voices commented to him about what was going on. Loosening of associations, delusions, and hallucinations led to the diagnosis of schizophrenia. As Jacob did not respond to antipsychotic medication, he was not discharged.

Using the NeuroAnalysis framework it is clear that Jacob's major problem is related to connectivity breakdown in his brain. The normal connectivity among brain units and the activity of brain states allows for a coherent, consistent, and adaptable experience of the real world. Jacob's experience gradually became fragmented, incoherent, and illogical, and consequently included false reconciliations with false conclusions and interpretations of the world.

When brain states act independently without connecting constraints the global brain trajectory disintegrates and begins to jump from one state to an unrelated state, disintegrating associations. Combinations that would not have occurred had the system remained stably connected now take place. Thus unrelated events and ideas recombine and produce a "meaningful" connection. This is how strange, illogical ideas emerge and cause delusions.

Integration of multimodal systems also suffers disconnection (see previous chapters); thus language processing and related auditory processing brain systems can act independently, allowing voices and speech to be generated even when there is no auditory input or visual correlates. This allows voices to be heard when there are no external sources of speech.

Medications do not help Jacob and do not relieve him of the

consequences of this disorganized activity. We do not really know how antipsychotic agents act on neural connectivity to enable resumption of functional connectivity. As for reconnecting cortical brain regions, perhaps in the future combined plasticity, inducing medication, and controlled cortical activation procedures (e.g., TMS and DBS) will enable controlled synchronized activation of auditory brain systems together with other relevant processes, by "relinking" connections and balancing brain processes to eliminate hallucinations.

If applied to the relevant disconnections in Jacob's brain, reorganization may cure his delusions and loosening of associations. This would not be an easy task. First, the exact algorithm of breakdown in the millisecond range time scale will have to be decoded. Then millisecond range synchronization would need to be effectuated and probably synchronized with specific cognitive challenges relevant to the systems that need controlling and reconnecting.

Using brain profiling evaluation, it is evident that the major (and probably only) problem in Jacob's brain relates to neural complexity disorder (NCD) of the segregated type (Figure 7.1). The smaller graph within Jacob's diagram shows a high score of connectivity imbalance in comparison with hierarchical imbalance that remains low.

Benjamin

Benjamin is a 55-year-old schizophrenia patient who resides in a hostel. For the past ten years his diagnosis was schizophrenia, residual type. He is a very isolated and quiet patient. Benjamin never talks spontaneously and utters only a few words when approached. If asked to talk about his feelings or experiences he is not able to elaborate. He typically responds with "yes" or "no" and, if asked about more complex situations, he answers, "don't know" or "don't remember."

Benjamin's facial expression is always blunt and does not reveal emotions. This does not change when he talks and even when conditions are supposed to be pleasant for him (e.g., family visits and so on). At times he wears a silly, smiling expression, often without any correlated external event. He sleeps a lot and if he is not woken in the morning he would probably spend the entire day in bed. Getting up is a tough ceremony overcome with great difficulty. He may usually be found lying on the grass or in the garden near the hostel.

Benjamin was not always like that; his medical records show that although he was not a bright student, he graduated from high school and had a decent job. Then suddenly he started to behave strangely. He failed at work and was fired, and he became tense and irritated. He talked to himself and neglected his personal hygiene. He would not sleep at nights and would take long walks in the streets.

As his disorder began to emerge, his parents, becoming increasingly concerned, brought him to the doctor who immediately referred him to a psychiatrist. Benjamin was diagnosed with a psychotic episode after the psychiatric evaluation revealed that he heard voices and had ideas of reference of control and thought insertions. He was convinced that aliens from outer space had taken control of his body and spirit, and were controlling his every thought and action. In addition, his thoughts were transmitted worldwide and were apparent to everyone on the globe. The aliens talked to him using human voices, commenting on every move he made. Antipsychotic agents administered in the psychiatric outpatient clinic largely reduced the intrusive thoughts and voices; however, the voices never completely disappeared, and kept coming back when he stopped taking his medication.

Once antipsychotic medications ameliorated his disturbing thoughts and voices, other problems arose. He felt drained, lost his willpower, and nothing interested him any more. Benjamin felt as if he was outside of events and that what happened around him was not related to him, as if he was observing life through a glass window. He was no longer interested in people or things. Even the affection he had always felt for his parents was gone and he regarded them as strangers. He was drawn to bed, and he had no reason to get up. He could not bring himself to go to work; the tasks at work seemed unimportant and dull. His general attitude was total disregard. When he was finally fired it was a relief and he did not care.

Assuming that his medications were the source of his weakness and inefficacy he stopped taking them, hoping to feel better without them. Once off medication he gradually started to experience an alien takeover. He began hearing voices again, tension grew, and it was only a matter of time before he was taken to the psychiatrist again.

This pattern repeated itself over and over again, and with each new episode his condition deteriorated until he needed intensive daily care. His parents finally admitted him to a hostel, realizing that they could no longer cope with his deteriorating condition. As the years went by while living in the hostel he took his medications under staff supervision, and they helped reduce his psychotic episodes but did not affect the deterioration which continued and ultimately left him totally incapacitated.

What happened to Benjamin? If we adopt the NeuroAnalysis approach then we can assume that the connectivity dynamics that normally matures at adolescence did not reach the level required for coping with the complexity of adult life. There are many possible explanations for this; perhaps biochemical processes of neural adhesion and synaptic growth were impaired. Alternatively, perhaps experience-dependent plasticity was induced via nurturing in the developmental years, and family influences were delayed or inadequate.

Whatever the reason, during early adulthood his brain suffered a connectivity imbalance strong enough to create a "segregated" type perturbation that fragmented his conscious experience and allowed delusions and hallucinations to take over his daily experience. Assuming that the optimization and homeostasis dynamics characteristic of the brain would initiate integration dynamics to counteract the effects of segregation in the brain, overconnectivity patterns of integration could take over the brain dynamics. Once over-integration occurs, brain states are fixated to a few constricted states and the global dynamic organization becomes limited, resulting in a marked reduction of all neural computations. Thoughts are restricted and orientation to the incoming events from the outer world is not met with responses. The hierarchical organization of the brain becomes deficient because global brain organization fails to organize at higher levels of transmodal systems. These systems become deficient and the emergent property they promote (i.e., volition) is reduced. This explains the sensation of abulia described in Benjamin's experience, abulia that steadily increased from one psychotic episode to the other.

This increase of abulia reflects the continuous deterioration of higher level organization within transmodal brain systems, and causes deficient hierarchal organization with higher level formations abolished and with a bottom-up insufficiency type of connectivity imbalance (see previous chapters and Figure 5.1).

Figure 7.1 shows that in Benjamin's case the impairment in his brain is with the NCD. Thus Benjamin's general brain profile is quite similar to Jacob's. However, in Benjamin's case the high NCD scores originate from scoring high on hierarchical imbalance, specifically bottom-up insufficiency, and not connectivity balance as is typical of Jacob's disturbance.

Samuel

Samuel is a 45-year-old widower with six children. He was hospitalized for approximately four months for a court-ordered forensic evaluation after he was arrested for driving without a license. In the hospital Samuel developed a depressive reaction with agitation and suicidal ideation, which extended his hospitalization for treatment purposes.

His family was of low socioeconomic status, and he attended school only through grade five. He spent most of his time on the streets with other children from similar backgrounds. Samuel still has trouble reading and writing. As a child he was impulsive, easily irritated, and had very low frustration levels. He was frequently involved in street fights and petty theft. He used some street drugs but did not become an addicted user.

At age 18 he got his driving license and started working as a truck driver, and later as a bus driver. He liked to drive, and earned enough to make ends meet. But even though he could work, he had difficulty holding a steady job, and adapting to a routine necessary for working in a trucking or bus company. He would typically get fired for not showing up on time, or being irresponsible – for example, changing driving routes and schedules. He had an all-or-nothing attitude and, if he was criticized by his boss even for minor problems, he would angrily quit his job.

Samuel eventually married and had children. The responsibility of having a family encouraged him to try and keep a steady job and he ultimately succeeded. His family described him as a lively person, though childish, irresponsible, impulsive and easily angered, frustrated, and depressed. He was indecisive and needed others to tell him what to do. After he got married, his wife assumed that responsibility and helped him to succeed in holding a job.

One day while driving his bus on a dark road he hit a motorcycle in a head-on collision. The two riders on the motorcycle died in the accident and he was taken in for questioning by the police. His driving license was permanently revoked.

Without his license he could not work. Employment attempts at factories or other menial tasks failed, and he remained unemployed. This created great stress for him as his already difficult financial situation plunged even further and he could not provide for his family.

In addition, his wife was diagnosed with cancer and died soon after. Samuel became a single parent, with no moral support and no financial capabilities. He reacted with a depressed mood that quickly turned into a major depression. He was depressed all the time, stopped eating, lost weight, isolated himself, and neglected his physical needs and personal hygiene. He became desperate, and when he started talking about killing himself he was taken to the doctor who referred him to a psychiatric hospital.

Samuel's medical records reveal that during his first hospitalization he had thoughts that his family and the medical staff were conspiring to lock him up and harm him. He was convinced that other patients were planning to kill him. Thus, in addition to his depressive symptoms he was diagnosed with delusions of persecution. The medical records showed a lack of consensus regarding his diagnosis. It appeared at times that he had major depressive disorder and at other times he was diagnosed with schizoaffective disorder. The paranoid ideation was considered part of a schizophreniform disorder and, together with the depressive clinical manifestation, he met diagnostic criteria for schizoaffective disorder.

Samuel's paranoid thinking resolved soon after he began antipsychotic pharmacotherapy. With the addition of antidepressant medication, his depressive symptoms ameliorated as well. He was discharged and soon after stopped coming to the outpatient clinic. He managed without any medication and adapted to his new situation at home. With the help of the municipal social welfare department he was able to manage and get on with his life.

As mentioned above, his current hospitalization was due to the judge's request for a forensic opinion. Even though at the start of the evaluation there were no signs and symptoms, within hours he met criteria for the diagnoses of depression and psychosis. His prior diagnostic entities emerged and he was diagnosed with schizoaffective disorder. He was declared unable to stand trial and was involuntarily admitted to a psychiatric institution due to suicidal risk and psychosis.

In Samuel's case the mental conditions that required hospitalization were clearly reactive in nature. They corresponded with stressful life events. In the first case it was the combined stress of losing his job, involvement in a fatal traffic accident, and losing his wife (who was evidently a supportive figure for him) to cancer. Many people endure similar tragic and stressful life events, but do not end up hospitalized with depressive and psychotic clinical conditions. Why did Samuel react as he did? What are Samuel's personality traits, coping capacities, and psychological strengths?

From Samuel's personal history it is evident that he had trouble developing a mature, durable, and adaptive personality structure. He typically suffered from low frustration levels. He was impulsive, unstable, and irrational throughout most of his young adulthood. He stabilized after receiving continuous support from his wife, but when she died he quickly lost control. Community welfare agencies stepped in, offered social support, and helped Samuel readjust, and thus averted the re-emergence of clinical symptoms.

Samuel's major "weakness" stems from inadequacies related to his personality development. The clinical presentations in the episodes described reflect reactions or perturbations to the already weak organization levels of his personality. Personality disorder (of some immature type) rather than schizoaffective disorder (as DSM-related diagnosis tends to suggest) should be his primary diagnosis, and the additional symptoms should be viewed as expressions of a decompensated mental system confronted with stressful events.

Using the NeuroAnalysis theoretical framework, it is evident that organizing factors necessary for development in early childhood were lacking. As a result his brain system may have suffered early-stage organization insufficiency. As a consequence, internal representations of the outer world remained partially developed, connectivity structures partially formed, and the entire system vulnerable to perturbation connectivity and optimization shifts (see previous chapters). These deficits were expressed behaviorally and emotionally by immature impulsive altitudes. For example, all-or-nothing impulsive reactions may be the expression of partial incomplete attractor formation, and thus incomplete and partial internal representations (of objects). Emotionally he easily became anxious and depressed, pointing to a disorder of optimization dynamics in his brain. The developmental deficiencies of childhood probably left him with deficient neuronal resilience and a neural resilience insufficiency (NRI) spread out in his neural network brain formations.

Once destabilized, optimization shifts emerged as mood swings, irritation, anxiety, and depression. When this dynamic shift increases, constraints among neural brain units and neural processes may disconnect, breaking down the normal connectivity balances in the brain. When this connectivity imbalance is severe enough, associations break down, new meanings that are unrelated to actual events and evidence from the real outer world occurrences can emerge. For example, hospitalization, intended to promote Samuel's care and protection, was distorted in his understanding, and experienced as menacing and persecuting.

Charting his clinical condition according to the brain profiling schema (Figure 7.1) it is evident that his major problem is context-sensitive processing decline (CSPD), as explained above, due to his deficient personality maturation. The NRI (neural reliance insufficiency) is scored next as very high; the tendency to collapse connectivity formations and balances is marginal and thus scored lowest.

Tim

Tim is a 35-year-old divorcee living with his parents. He has one child who is now living with his former wife, the mother. A year ago he was badly injured in a car accident while driving home from work. A car that was heading in the opposite direction deviated from its course and hit his car head-on.

Tim suffered multi-system injuries including a head injury that involved a skull fracture. He was found unconscious outside of his car, which overturned from the impact of the collision. He was treated by ambulance paramedics on the scene, and then taken to the emergency room. A CAT-scan performed in the emergency room revealed massive intracranial hemorrhage and contusions to the left and right frontal hemispheres.

After extended hospitalization, when he gradually regained consciousness he was sent to a rehabilitation center. During his first weeks in rehabilitation he was confused, did not recognize his family, and did not remember anything about his past. He was irritated and agitated and needed heavy sedation.

Gradually he started to regain his orientation in time and began recognizing people, but he still had difficulty organizing his thinking and actions. This was evident from his tendency to speak in a very erratic manner, jumping from one subject to another. At times he exhibited "word salad" (i.e., consecutively used words that were not related).

He was very concrete and took everything literally. When he was asked what had brought him to the hospital (meaning what was wrong with him) he would say "the blue bus." However, Tim's most serious problem was controlling his temper and urges, among others his sexual urges. He had outbursts where he shouted and even became violent. He could not tolerate delaying satisfaction and wanted immediate responses to his demands. He made provocative and inappropriate sexual advances to staff nurses. This behavior made his management very difficult and seriously hampered efforts to promote his rehabilitation.

Medications ameliorated these behaviors well enough to have him discharged. Back home his family experienced him as a totally different man than he was before the accident. He was described as very childish, insecure, and easily irritated. When he did not receive immediate satisfaction of his needs, even the smallest disturbance could trigger a rampage. He could not work or concentrate on any task for more then a few minutes and his understanding was seriously hampered due to his concrete views.

Tim was discharged from hospital with two diagnoses, both related to "head injury." The first was "cognitive impairment due to brain damage." This diagnosis was based on consecutive brain imaging examinations showing he was left with bilateral frontal lobe cortical atrophy and probably also a widespread demyelination axonal injury (DAI) due to massive edema that followed the brain concussion. The second diagnosis was "organic personality disorder"; this was based on his behavior and change in personality. In fact, this change was so dramatic that he actually became a different person from the man his wife had married and lived with before the accident. Due to these changes and the consequent behaviors his wife divorced him and he went back to live with his parents.

Using the NeuroAnalysis perspective we must consider the effects of a massive loss of neural networks both globally and specifically in the frontal cortices. Neuroscience has explained the critical importance of the frontal lobes for our intellectual and mental higher functions. In effect the frontal lobe is involved in almost all of the cognitive functions. It is especially relevant for higher level cognitive functions such as abstract reasoning and decision-making. It is also relevant to cognitive adaptation set-shifting and focusing attention on complex tasks.

We also know much about the inhibitory effect of the frontal-lobe functions (specifically orbito-frontal cortices) on urges and drives. Releasing these inhibitions accounts for inappropriate sexual behavior and non-adaptive low frustration rates. These result in the outbursts and near-violent episodes characterizing Tim's behavior (see above).

Going back to NeuroAnalysis, in general, the loss of neural network structure reduces all neural computation capabilities in the brain. More specifically the loss of fronto-orbital and frontal-lobe neural networks represents a loss of higher level brain organization. The frontal lobe, if functional, is a high-connectivity system with massive efferent and afferent connections with all brain regions and systems. As such it is the grand coordinator and organizer of most if not all of the brain's activity. With this major organizing function debilitated, the brain is left "uncoordinated" and thus "untuned" to computational demand. Neural networks may act in disharmony, allowing for brain states to be activated independently without any correlation or constraint among themselves, and thus can explain the loosening of associations that initially characterized Tim's condition.

More serious is the lack of higher level network systems of the brain hierarchy; the frontal lobe is one of the transmodal brain systems (see previous chapters) and without such systems conscious experience may be hampered and reduced. This may explain the initial confusion and lack of orientation described in Tim's clinical history. Furthermore, the transmodal systems imbed the configurational attractor systems that allow for internal representations of the outer psychosocial world. These are the internal representations (or object representations), which govern our way of perceiving and reacting to psychosocial events. This is what determines the expression of our personality traits.

It is obvious then that if this is disturbed then the expression of personality will be altered. If the internal representation of the world (of objects) becomes damaged it can become less complex, less differentiated, and lacking; thus it reverses and becomes analogous to primitive immature primordial internal configurations, similar to those of the undeveloped infant and child. As such it is comprehensible why Tim's behavior resembled the immature behavior of a child.

Deficient higher levels are also responsible for the lack of top-down processes in the brain hierarchy. These top-down processes that regulate and inhibit up-coming hierarchical processes enable us to act on the basis of context representations and higher levels of consideration for many aspects of the complex environment. When these functions are missing, goal-planning decision-making and thinking order is disturbed.

Taking into consideration the types of dynamic alterations to the widespread brain organization, the lack of controlled hierarchal connectivity as well as general balanced connectivity, the unstable optimization shifts and constraint frustration typically explain the tension and rage that easily occur.

Tim's diagram in Figure 7.1 shows the massive deficits that involve al three brain profiling axes: the NCD, the NRI, and the CSPD. All three have similarly high scores. This means that neural complexity, neural resilience, and context-sensitive processing are all deficient. The two smaller graphs within Tim's diagram represent the factors that make up the scores of the three major scales. To the right is the graph of two factors that contribute to the NCD. These are the connectivity imbalance and the hierarchical imbalance. Both are high, as is evident in the graph. The sub-graph on the left represents the contributors for the NRI scale. They are the "optimization imbalance" and the "constraint frustration imbalance," they too have high values, especially the "constraint frustration imbalance."

These graphs represent the brain profiling of Tim and can provide for his diagnosis when the causes of this description are also added and explained. Actually it is evidence of massive brain damage involving all aspects of brain organization.

John

John is 40 years old, married, and has three children. In the past five years he has been hospitalized in a closed psychiatric ward due to severe changes in behavior, specifically violent behavior directed toward both others and himself. His medical record shows no special psychiatric history. Five years ago he was treated with benzodiazepines following complaints of an anxious mood due to pressures at work. He responded well to the treatment and took his medications regularly. He sometimes increased the dosages of his medications without informing his doctor in an attempt to cope better with the stressors at work.

After a year of treatment his doctor noticed that John was increasing his dosage extensively and that the medication was getting out of hand. Owing to the potential withdrawal effects of benzodiazepines, the physician instructed John to taper down the dosage according to a treatment plan to gradually stop the medications. The plan to take him off these meds was successful.

A few weeks after stopping his treatment, John began having episodes of confusion. His wife described him as becoming perplexed, as if he did not recognize his whereabouts. These episodes could last for thirty minutes to an hour. During that time he would talk nonsense, unrelated to the conversation that was going on. He also suddenly became silent and disconnected for a few seconds as if he was unaware of his surroundings. On these occasions, when approached, he would respond as if snapping out of a daydream.

As time passed these episodes became frequent and longer; they were also accompanied by irritable behavior which increased gradually. By now John was on sick leave from work and under medical investigation for his behavior. As part of his medical investigation he was referred to a psychiatrist who recommended commencing low-dose antipsychotic medication. Despite the treatment his condition deteriorated and one day, after breaking up furniture at home and endangering his family, he was hospitalized.

Once hospitalized, he was diagnosed as suffering from a psychotic episode and put on an increased dosage of antipsychotics. John had become quite violent, to the extent that he needed frequent restraint and seclusion. His wife told the medical staff that he had changed radically and was not the same person she married and knew before. She anxiously asked the treating physicians what had happened to her husband. At this point several diagnostic entities were considered by his psychiatrist. The prevailing diagnosis was schizophrenia or schizophreniform psychosis.

Not all members of the staff agreed with this diagnosis and the young resident psychiatrist directly responsible for his care had some serious doubts. The resident had just learned that schizophrenia psychosis typically starts at an earlier age and that it often involves auditory hallucinations and/or delusions of reference or of persecution. The resident psychiatrist also learned that schizophrenia patients sometimes become violent in response to the content of their delusions.

In John's case violence seemed to be aimless and unrelated to any delusion; in effect he did not report any hallucinations and did not exhibit hallucinatory behavior. Even though a senior psychiatrist in the department tended to interpret his episodes of absence as hallucinatory behavior, the interpretation was not definitive and was not supported by the patient's complaints. In addition, his psychosis started at a late age not typical to classic schizophrenia onset.

Even though the diagnosis of schizophrenia became a consensus in the department, John's resident psychiatrist was not convinced by this diagnosis, and his doubts increased as John did not respond to treatment. Instead of becoming better with treatment, the opposite occurred. When dosages were increased and the type of antipsychotic medication was changed, his condition worsened, and it seemed that worsening was correlated with the treatment itself.

As time progressed, additional staff members began to question the diagnosis. The doubts increased when John's condition worsened and he began to reveal "organic" symptoms. He was frequently confused, initially not being aware of the date and time, and later on he lost his sense of space, and did not know where his room was located. He began to confuse people with others, and referred to his psychiatrist as though she was his wife.

Furthermore, when placed in seclusion following a violent episode, he started to lose control over his sphincter and smeared his feces on the walls and door of the seclusion room. This behavior, together with loss of orientation and confusion, was clearly taking him toward the diagnosis of some "organic" brain disorder. A neurological investigation including brain imaging was initiated. Disappointingly however, both his CT and MRI (magnetic resonance imaging) showed no brain injury. John was diagnosed with organic brain psychosis, he did not respond to antipsychotic medication, and his daily treatment involved frequent restraints and seclusions. An ECT (electro-convulsive treatment) trial proved temporarily beneficial, but the effect of the treatment was short and lasted for only a few hours after every treatment session.

Just as the prognosis of John's case seemed to worsen and his psychiatrists became very discouraged, his resident psychiatrist stumbled on a clinical entity that may explain John's case. While preparing for the neurology examination in his residency program, he learned about the medical diagnosis of Nonconvulsive Status Epilepticus (NCSE). The mental status changes reported in NCSE may be subtle to the degree that only family or friends notice them, or they may manifest as marked changes in behavior, psychosis, and even coma. The variety of clinical presentations includes speech disturbance, which can vary from verbal perseveration to aphasia, to cognitive disturbances that can affect attention, memory, or both. The cognitive disturbances can be mild or result in prolonged confusional states. Affective and psychotic changes have also been described and are sometimes confused with primary psychiatric illnesses. Frequently, fluctuations in the clinical presentation make diagnosis difficult. Automatisms, myoclonic jerks, abnormal motor activity, and eye twitching or deviation may be minimally present, although motor activity is normal in most cases.

It is important to emphasize that patients with NCSE can appear to be functioning "normally" and that manifestations of the status may be as subtle as decreased attention or slight clumsiness; therefore, when the patient or family observes that the patient is not at baseline, it should raise suspicion and prompt an investigation.

Because of the wide range of clinical presentations, lack of or minimal motor activity, and fluctuation of symptoms, it is easy to understand how the diagnosis of NCSE can be missed or confused with a psychiatric disorder or nonepileptic neurologic disorder. A detailed history including past medical conditions, social history, medications, and changes in medications is essential. The history should include information from family members or caregivers whenever possible.

Information about changes from baseline, onset and duration of the events, presence or absence of postictal symptoms, and presence or absence of fluctuating symptoms all help to develop the differential diagnosis. A history of a seizure disorder, especially when the patient's symptoms are temporally related to a convulsive event, is a red flag that needs to be investigated. Prolonged postictal periods or persisting aphasic, somatosensory, or psychic findings after the ictus should raise suspicions of possible ongoing epileptogenic activity.

It was not an easy task to have this patient do an EEG (electroencephalography) examination, due to his erratic behavior. Nevertheless, the examination was partly successful, and although results were not fully indicative of epileptic activity some slow waves dispersal in the frontal cortical regions suggested that some seizure EEG activity may have been taking place in his brain. Consequently he was immediately taken off his antipsychotic medication (known to increase epileptic risk by lowering neural seizure activity) and put on anticonvulsive therapy.

The improvement was immediate, John's confusion disappeared, and he became much more organized. He later regained most of his premorbid capability. He was finally able to be discharged to go back home and try to resume his previously normal life. He never achieved the same capabilities as before his illness and had to cope with mild cognitive impairment that fluctuated somewhat over the years.

Using the NeuroAnalysis formulations, what transpired in John's brain was a disturbance to the threshold function of neurons. Neurons have an input–output regulation which occurs via threshold mechanisms in each neuron (see previous neural computation sections). Activity of neural network ensembles are balanced not solely by connectivity function (as described previously) but also by threshold functions; if threshold are reduced, neurons will become sensitive to inputs firing even at low-level inputs. These alterations can cause neural circuits to elicit excessive electrical activity within connected neural circuits. These circuits not only fall out of regular information-processing activity but they also interfere with process-triggering computations (i.e., actions, ideations, recognitions) that are removed from any environmentally dependent computation, thus throwing conscious activity into a realm of bias and aberrations. These biases appear clinically in the form of the disturbances described in John's case above.

The antipsychotic medication, known to increase seizure activity, worsened John's condition by further reducing the threshold values in his neural network units. The ECT treatment was beneficial temporarily because it is known to increase neuronal threshold functions. Finally, anticonvulsive therapy which probably acts by normalizing threshold levels had the best therapeutic effect on John's brain.

Brain profiling is not directly relevant to John's case as it is not directly relevant to neurological (non-psychiatric) phenomena. In essence John's brain disturbance is of the neural complexity type, and thus there are NCD scores only. The reduced neuronal threshold function caused a general disturbance to the interrelation among neuronal ensembles and is thus similar to a connectivity alteration spread in the cortex both hierarchically and generally.

Daniel

Daniel is a 42-year-old engineer, married with two children. Four years ago he had his first encounter with a psychiatric clinic after he suffered severe depression. His depression began very gradually at first; he felt tired and weak, especially during the weekends. He attributed this to his demanding job and he hoped it would pass if he had enough rest. However, as it grew worse he went to his family practitioner who ordered a blood count and blood chemistry, and had him checked over physically. As his results were normal he was told to rest or take a vacation.

Over the next few weeks things became worse. He began to feel moody, sad most of the day, felt no initiative at work, and in effect everything he did became difficult. He was not sleeping well, woke up a few times during the night, and finally got up earlier than required, being unable to complete his night's sleep. He lost his appetite and started to lose weight. He noticed the weight loss when his clothes suddenly felt large. Worst of all was his mindset. He started to see everything in a pessimistic and hopeless manner, and finally began to believe that he would be better off dead. He did not want to commit suicide but he found himself wishing for an accident that would cause his death and relieve him from his condition. He began to receive letters from his supervisors at work, warning him that he was not doing his job properly.

Daniel's wife was concerned by his talk of getting killed, and worried about his generally deteriorating condition. She contacted a psychiatrist recommended by a friend and made an appointment for Daniel. The psychiatrist made a clear-cut diagnosis of Major Depressive Disorder according to the DSM diagnostic method. Daniel filled the criteria for major depression, depressed mood, insomnia, weight loss and reduced appetite, suicidal ideation, despair and hopelessness, and so on.

Selective serotonin reuptake inhibitors (SSRIs) are a set of anti-depressant medications effective in treating depression. Daniel responded to this treatment, and after two weeks on this SSRI medication he improved, and after another three weeks he was in full remission and back to his old self. After the first depressive episode, under the supervision of his psychiatrist, Daniel stopped his medication, hoping it was a single passing depressive episode. However, six months later a new episode emerged. The second time it took longer to pass and Daniel was put on a maintenance dose of antidepressants which prevented recurring depressive episodes until recently.

The recent depressive episode emerged six months ago and began while Daniel was on his maintenance dose. Reviewing his case notes, Daniel's psychiatrist noticed that his medical work-up was not complete; thyroid hormone and adrenaline hormone levels were not evaluated. Daniel was sent immediately for a full medical checkup and, as suspected by his psychiatrist, his laboratory test results revealed a serious reduction of thyroid hormone levels. Medication to correct Daniel's thyroid hormonal levels proved effective immediately, and his depressive episode passed. SSRI medication was stopped, and with balanced thyroid function it seemed that the depression was not coming back. Daniel's psychiatrist concluded that his depression was due to hypothyroidism and determined a favorable prognosis providing he adhere to his thyroid medication to maintain normal thyroid levels.

If we examine Daniel's story from the NeuroAnalysis theoretical point of view, we may assume that neural network systems in his brain suffered reduced neural resilience due to a deficiency in the thyroid hormone. Currently it is unknown how the thyroid hormone reduces neural resilience; however, it is apparent that many hormones effect neuronal activity and some are also defined as neurohormones.

Once massive deficits in neural resilience occurred in Daniel's brain, his neural network systems became ineffective for the computations needed to maintain his brain activity effectively. His neural network systems began having difficulty optimizing functions and representations. Instead of optimizing attractor systems in the brain these remained deoptimized. As deoptimization dynamics increased, the emergent property of depressed mood appeared (see emergent properties in previous chapters).

SSRIs are known to increase neural resilience (see previous chapters). By doing so they counterbalanced the deficiency caused by inadequate levels of thyroid hormone, enabling a remission from depressive symptoms. Figure 7.1 shows Daniel's brain profiling pattern; the NRI (Neuronal Resilience Insufficiency) score is obviously high, and deoptimization shift (not constraint frustration) is the major contributor to this disturbance.

Figure 7.3 shows the clinician's chart of evaluation in the case of Daniel. The marked circles show the clinical findings and the marked square proposes that deoptimization is the cause of his brain disturbance.

In comparison to David's (the first patient) chart it is evident that in Daniel's case the disturbance is limited to the level of optimization dynamics with connectivity and constraints levels conserved.

Sandra

Sandra, aged 32, was admitted to the emergency room of a general hospital after ingesting an overdose of sedative medication in an attempt to commit suicide. After regaining consciousness she was referred to a psychiatric consultation in the emergency room. Her psychiatric interview revealed that her suicide attempt was the result of overwhelming feelings of worthlessness and depression. These feelings had built up rapidly during the weekend and by Sunday evening she felt that there was nothing to live for any more.

A careful investigation beyond her complaints regarding the symptoms of depression and feelings of worthlessness revealed a complicated picture involving a relevant, meaningful relationship she was

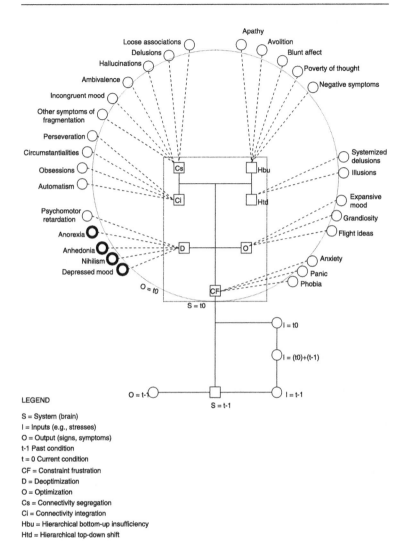

Figure 7.3 Daniel's clinical evaluation.

having with her boyfriend. Her feelings of desolation and despair began at the beginning of the weekend when her boyfriend cancelled plans to spend the weekend together; instead, he drove out of town to spend the weekend with his mother. Sandra understood and agreed, but soon after she began to feel frustrated, angry, and alone.

She felt that she was not worthy of her boyfriend's attention and care. She felt rejected and useless.

In the emergency room her treatment was for "crises intervention," she had no psychotic symptoms, and no symptoms of major depression. Her depressive episode was short (limited to the two days of the weekend) and, during her twenty-four-hour stay in the emergency room she recovered, her feelings of despair dissipated, and with them the suicidal ideation passed.

A second checkup by the psychiatrist found no justification for hospitalization and she was referred to the outpatient clinic for follow-up and psychological intervention as continued care related to crisis intervention. She was discharged from the emergency room with the diagnosis of "adjustment reaction."

At the outpatient clinic she was scheduled for a psychological evaluation. Her personal history unfolded during that evaluation. At the age of 1, she was taken away from her mother and sent to an orphanage. She remained in the orphanage until she was adopted at age 3. She never found out why her mother had to give her up and she was planning to open up her adoption files once she had gained the courage to do so. She had very few memories of her early childhood at the orphanage, and remembered mainly the constant turnover of caregivers who were always busy taking care of all of the children in the crowded institution. She remembered that for the first time she felt the attention and warmth of home when she reached her adoptive family. Even though from age 3 she was raised in a very supportive, loving environment she always felt that she was not good enough, and needed attention and compliments to feel worthy and esteemed. Growing up, she was very sensitive to the opinions of others; for example, at school she was known to be a very "sensitive" student. If a teacher or her peers criticized her, even in a minor way, Sandra's reactions were extreme and she became disproportionately angry or depressed.

Her relationships were unstable with her peers; she never had a special, enduring friendship. Sandra often initiated relationships with enthusiasm, investing everything in the friendship, but she quickly grew fed up and ended the relationship. Thus her interpersonal relationships were typically accompanied by feelings of enthusiasm and elation at first, and dissolution and depression at the end. Thus both her social relationships as well as her moods were characterized by shifts and instability.

As a young adult this type of behavior characterized her relationships with men. She changed partners frequently. She was generally overly enthusiastic at the beginning of a relationship, and quite depressed when the relationship ended.

At the psychiatric interview in the emergency room she described her recent relationship with her current boyfriend as a repetition of her typical relationships. When she met him and first fell in love with him he was the perfect person, though she told the psychiatrist that he had many problems, including a history of trouble with the law. She was blind to his faults. However, when he went to visit his mother and left her alone for the weekend, he suddenly seemed to become an awful person and she detested him. She told the psychiatrist that she was determined to end her relationship with him immediately.

This information about problems with interpersonal relationships (and the absence of depression or psychosis) supported the diagnosis of personality disorder. As expected, these unstable, interpersonal relationships were not limited to personal friendships but also extended to her occupational history. The psychiatric interview revealed frequent job changes. She never held a steady job for more than eighteen months. The in-depth interview revealed that most of the time Sandra was the one who quit, generally following minor criticism by her boss. Even if she was instructed about some job requirement that to the psychiatrist seemed normal for any work setting, it implied criticism to Sandra. She was quick to decide that she could not go on like that, that the workplace was not good for her career, and so she would quit.

The clinic was a public university teaching outpatient clinic where she was assigned to a resident psychologist who was being trained and supervised in this case. As expected, her initial attitude toward the therapist was very good; she felt she had received the best therapist in the clinic and that he was the perfect practitioner. At the beginning of therapy the therapist collected the initial information for his psychotherapeutic evaluation. The encounter was characterized by many questions and a lot of attention from the therapist. The attention generated in Sandra feelings of elation, as she was the center of attention and this made her feel important and valuable. Her self-esteem was boosted and the first psychotherapeutic encounters were characterized by a marked improvement in mood energies and motivations.

The therapist had collected the information relevant for him to predict what would transpire next. He was aware that her interpersonal relationships tended to topple and invert; this was predicted to occur in the therapeutic setting because psychotherapy is also an interpersonal relationship, and as such it is similar to other interpersonal attitudes outside of therapy settings. However, as he was an inexperienced resident, he was not prepared for the switch to happen so fast and for no readily apparent reason.

At the fifth meeting Sandra told her therapist about her intentions to open her adoption files to find out the identity of her birth parents. The therapist, curious about the procedure for revealing adoption information, asked Sandra what was involved. Her response was sharp and abrupt, reflecting a dramatic change in her attitude toward her therapist. "What kind of therapist are you if you do not know about such procedures?" she asked angrily. The therapist saw her as never before, angry, hurt, and distant.

The therapist who a moment ago was the best professional now suddenly seemed to Sandra to be incapable and incompetent. This feeling was accompanied by great distress because she felt she deserved the best, and that with such an incompetent therapist she was probably not worthy of proper attention, meaning that she was worthless.

At supervision the therapist learned to apply psychotherapeutic theories to this case. Partial object representations, the splitting of object and self-representation with the splitting expressed as idealization/devaluation was relevant to what had been happening in the therapeutic meetings.

Due to her early life experiences, and lacking the normal support for proper development, Sandra probably had difficulty developing the differentiations needed for good early object representations. As described by theoreticians such as Kernberg (1978), the internal representations of the self–object and the internalized external objects were not integrated, tending to stay "split" into "good" and "bad" opposing positive and negative representations; thus meaningful others can be either "all good" (idealized) or "all bad" (devaluated). There is a kind of "blindness" to the complexity of others (i.e., having both positive and negative aspects).

This is evident from her tendency to idealize her boyfriend. At first she was unable to see his downside, including his previous problems. This is also evident from her devaluation of him the moment he left her for the weekend. This kind of "split perception" of the meaningful other is exactly what transpired during the therapy sessions; first, the therapist was "all-perfect" and then, after showing some lack of knowledge, he became totally incapable and worthless.

In addition to the immature split object representations there was also a lack of differentiation between the representation of the self and the internalized external objects. This was expressed through the lack of differentiation in the way the meaningful other was experienced and the way she experienced herself. For example, Sandra devalued her boyfriend for leaving her alone for the weekend, thus immediately feeling that she herself was worthless and unworthy. With the therapist the same thing happened again. When the therapist was idealized as "the best" she was also important and elated for having apparently been treated by the best therapist, but when the therapist was devaluated and perceived as incapable, she was correspondingly also unworthy for having such an awful therapist.

Using the NeuroAnalysis perspective, we have seen that object representations can be embedded in the brain as attractor systems within the space state of the brain organization. The landscape that such attractor systems shape is like an internal map of representations shaped by experience and outer world occurrences. This landscape is developed and matures based on experience-dependent plasticity and on the support of neurological tissue structure. In the case of Sandra it is obvious that her early experiences were unstable and awkward. This affected the experience-dependent plasticity of Sandra's brain organization at an early age and left it undeveloped to support the complex internal representation needed for a fuller appreciation of occurring real life complexities.

The undeveloped internal configuration is by definition unable to match the external complexities of the outer world. This non-fitting configuration is a continuous source for deoptimization dynamics, because the internal configuration is never fully activated by the environmental patterns of incoming information. This is the case especially when there is a significant mismatch; for example, unreal expectations from a "perfect boyfriend" are obviously not fulfilled in real life.

As described in previous chapters deoptimization dynamics result in an emergent property of depressed mood, explaining why Sandra's complaints were typically of depression. It was predictable that the mismatch between internal and external representations left Sandra victim to repeated mood shifts and affective instability as has typically been described for patients with personality disorders.

The clinical brain profiling (CBP) graph for Sandra can be of two types (see Sandra, (a) and (b), Figure 7.1). Sandra (a) is the clinical brain profiling of Sandra during the depressed episode and Sandra (b) is the clinical brain profiling when not depressed.

Barbara

Barbara, aged 30, was referred to a psychiatrist after a long failed treatment for flight phobia by her behavioral psychologist. After three weeks' medication with Paroxetine 20mg/day Barbara took her first symptom-free flight.

It all started when as a teenager Barbara flew for the first time by herself. She had flown with her family before, but at around the age of 18 she was sent to visit family in Europe and was flying alone as her family waited for her to arrive at the destination airport.

During that flight she fell asleep. Half-way into the flight there was a problem with the airplane and the pilot decided to land the aircraft ahead of destination to avoid any possible risks. He instructed the cabin crew to notify the passengers about early landing, and to explain that it was due to a minor problem and that there was no need for alarm. Some of the passengers who were sleeping were awoken by the announcement, and others, including Barbara, slept right through.

As the descent for landing began, the crew awakened the sleeping passengers to instruct them to fasten their seat belts, and repeated the information regarding the unscheduled landing. Barbara had been in a deep sleep, and when awakened she was startled and at first did not know where she was. When she understood that there was to be an unscheduled landing, her startled response was augmented by a fear that the plane may crash, together with the anxiety of landing in a foreign airport where her family would not be waiting to greet her. She was also anxious that her family would worry as to the whereabouts of the plane. Barbara's worries intensified, and as the plane landed she started to feel her heart beating rapidly. She was sweating but felt cold and shivered. The circling of the plane made her extremely nauseous, and as her discomfort mounted she felt suffocated and certain that she was going to die.

Barbara's feelings gradually tapered down after the plane landed. The passengers were led to a transit lounge to wait for the plane to be repaired. One of the cabin attendants noticed that Barbara was feeling ill and the airport physician was summoned. He gave her two pills: one to take under the tongue just before take-off and the other in case she felt poorly even after taking the first pill. When the flight continued to its destination she took the first pill and had no problems for the rest of the flight. On her way back from the vacation a similar sensation of panic started to emerge immediately after take-off, and she was able to overcome her fears on the flight back home only with the help of the additional pill. Thereafter any attempt to fly was immediately accompanied by similar attacks that she realized were caused by "panic." These panic attacks were not limited to boarding an airplane. They began to occur when going into an underground parking lot or crowded elevator. Any situation that felt like the closed, crowded, inescapable cabin triggered the panic attacks.

Barbara went to a psychologist who immediately identified her clinical description as a typical panic attack related to flight phobia or phobia from crowded, closed places. She was offered behavioral therapy of desensitization. This involved learning relaxation techniques to counteract the sensations of panic; for example, learning to breathe slowly to counteract the suffocating hyperpnoea of the panic attack, and to relax the muscles to counteract the tension during the panic attack. After mastering this technique she would then be exposed gradually (according to a predetermined scale of feared conditions), each time exercising the relaxation technique to counteract the panic attack. Barbara went up the fear scale, each time counteracting a more fearful situation, and the goal was the extinction of all fear from even the most fearful condition on the scale.

Barbara did not succeed in this treatment, even though she mastered the relaxation techniques when she was exposed to the various fear conditions. Even at lower fear conditions on the scale she would feel the panic attack again; furthermore, having felt the panic attack would strengthen it, making her situation worse. The psychologist understood that treatment was causing her condition to deteriorate and decided to refer her to a psychiatrist for pharmacotherapy. After three weeks of medication her symptoms were gone and she could board a plane again.

Even though the manifestation of phobia and panic attacks are well-known clinical entities, the exact pathological mechanisms underlying these signs and symptoms are not known. Many theories exist and some are psychoanalytic, as explained in previous chapters. In psychological terms fear and panic attacks are signals of unconscious contents threatening to become conscious, destabilizing ego integrity. Behaviorist psychologists have an entirely different explanation (theory): that of learned, or more precisely associational learning, were there is an association (as in paired stimuli) when the fear is paired with the phobic stimulus.

In this case, as in many other similar descriptions, there is a sense of a learned experience, suggesting that we are dealing with something similar to an association where the fear feelings were paired with the airplane condition of close, inescapable surroundings.

Using the NeuroAnalysis hypothesis, anxiety and panic attacks are emergent properties of a disturbance to the constraint-satisfaction organization within neural network systems in the brain. This formulation has been good at reconciling psychological and biological formulations in the explanation of anxiety disorders (see previous chapters). As explained, the perturbations to the constraint satisfaction among neutral network organization can be bound to a stimulus, in this case the stimulus of experiencing fear waking up in the airplane landing unexpectedly.

The event on the plane may be viewed as a constellation of situations that has generated a constellation-related input pattern to the brain via the specific constellation-related experience. This constellation-related pattern triggered a destabilization effect in the network system emerging as a sensation of panic and fear. Once the system was perturbed due to the specific constellation-related input patterns it became receptive to repeat the perturbation dynamics when a similar (not necessarily identical) constellation-related input pattern was introduced.

In Barbara's case her brain became "sensitive" to the constellation of a closed, inescapable place that was associated with some information of threat and fear. Consequently experiences that had similar constellations such as underground parking lots and closed elevators triggered a constraint-frustration dynamics spread in the brain, resulting in the emergent property of anxiety and fear.

The behavioral therapy did not succeed because every time she was exposed to an experience of similar constellation the constraint-frustration dynamics was triggered and strengthened. The medication, acting on the serotonin receptors by triggering second neurotransmitter activity and finally allowing synaptogenetic processes to take place, increased neural resilience. This resilience was achieved due to the increase of spines and dendrite connections allowing each neuron to be more reflexive in processing incoming and outgoing information. As such, the system as a whole is more flexible, allowing the constraints to become more flexible, further permitting the reduction of constraint frustration. The reduction of constraint frustrations allows for a better constraint-satisfaction dynamics, reducing the emergent property of fear and panic.

Using the CBP graph (Figure 7.1), Barbara's diagnostic profile shows high levels of neural resilience insufficiency (NRI) related to high levels of constraint-frustration imbalance.

Summary

This chapter of clinical examples starts out with a complicated patient, one whose symptoms are easily under-diagnosed using the traditional *Diagnostic and Statistical Manual* (DSM) approach. David scored high on all three dimensions of clinical brain profiling. Due to his history of developmental problems he scored high on context-sensitive process decline (CSPD); then, with destabilization of his system at the time of evaluation (S = t0 in Figure 7.2), he also scored high on many levels of disturbed brain organization including connectivity disturbances optimization and constraint-frustration levels.

This multifactor disturbance is not the case for the other patients. Jacob and Benjamin are patients with disturbance to connectivity organization limited either to the disconnection disturbance (Jacob) or hierarchical connectivity disturbances (Benjamin). Samuel's case is again more complex, involving developmental deficiency of the brain system with context-sensitive processing decline. However, in his case the destabilization of the system at the time of evaluation (hospitalizations) is related to the level of optimization resulting in a clinical picture of depression.

Tim's case exemplifies total damage to all brain organizations. In this case even though development of the system was achieved effectively, the damage is extensive to the degree that even the context-sensitive processing functions are destroyed.

Daniel's case is an example of a limited disturbance, limited in level and extent; it is limited to the level of optimization disturbances and to the extent of deoptimization alone. Daniel's case is a good example of the differences in presentation of the clinical chart between a simple, limited disturbance (Figure 7.3) and complex multilevel disturbances as in David's case (Figure 7.2).

Barbara's case is also limited in level and disturbance; it is limited to the level of disturbance to constraint frustration. In Sandra's case again, developmental problems of internal representations (contexts) and thus context-sensitive processing decline, making the picture of brain disorganization multilevel and more complex. Recurring deoptimizations and thus depressions occur.

The translation of clinical phenomena to the presumed brain disturbances has been exemplified here with the insight that this is only a preliminary attempt, and hopefully the beginning of a process that will lead to more effective translations that are necessary on the road toward unraveling the neurological origins of mental disorders.

References

Allen, R.M. and Young, S.J. (1978) Phencyclidine-induced psychosis. *American Journal of Psychiatry* 135: 1081–1084.

American Psychiatric Association (2000) *(DSM-IV-TR) Diagnostic and Statistical Manual of Mental Disorders*, 4th edn, text revision. Washington, DC: American Psychiatric Press, Inc.

Andreasen, N.C. (1983) *The Scale for the Assessment of Negative Symptoms (SANS)*. Iowa City: University of Iowa.

Andreasen, N.C. (1984) *The Scale for Assessment of Positive Symptoms (SAPS)*. Iowa City: University of Iowa.

Andreasen, N.C. (1997) Linking mind and brain in the study of mental illnesses: a project for a scientific psychopathology. *Science* 275: 1586–1596.

Andreasen, N.C. and Olsen, S. (1982) Negative and positive schizophrenia: definition and validation. *Archives of General Psychiatry* 39: 789–794.

Ariety, X. and Goldstein, K. (1959) *American Handbook of Psychiatry*. New York: Basic Books.

Baars, B.B. (1988) *A Cognitive Theory of Consciousness*. New York: Oxford University Press.

Barker, A.T., Jalinous, R., and Freeston, I.L. (1985) Noninvasive magnetic stimulation of the human motor cortex. *Lancet* 1(8437): 1106–1107.

Berking, C., Takemoto, R., Schaider, H., Showe, L., Satyamoorthy, K., Robbins, P., and Herlyn, M. (2001) Transforming growth factor-beta1 increases survival of human melanoma through stroma remodeling. *Cancer Research* 61: 8306–8316.

Bliss, T.V.P. and Gardner-Medwin, A.R. (1973) Long-lasting potentiation of synaptic transmission in the dentate area of the unanaesthetized rabbit following stimulation of the prefrontal path. *Journal of Physiology* 232: 357–374.

Brustein, E. and Rossignol, S. (1999) Recovery of locomotion after ventral and ventrolateral spinal lesions in the cat. II. Effects of noradrenergic and serotoninergic drugs. *Journal of Neurophysiology* 81: 1513–1530.

Cajal, S.R. (1911) *Histologie du Système Nerveux de L'homme et des Vertèbres*. Madrid: Institute Ramon y Cajal 1952 edn, Vol. 2. Madrid: Instituto Ramon y Cajal.

Cambel, A.B. (1993) *Applied Chaos Theory: A Paradigm for Complexity.* San Diego, CA: Academic Press.

Christiansen, C., Abreu, B., Ottenbacher, K., Huffman, K., Masel, B., and Culpepper, R. (1998) Task performance in virtual environments used for cognitive rehabilitation after traumatic brain injury. *Archives of Physical Medicine and Rehabilitation* 79: 888–892.

Cohen, J.D., Braver, T.S., and O'Reilly, R.C. (1996) A computational approach to prefrontal cortex, cognitive control and schizophrenia: recent developments and current challenges. *Philosophical Transactions of the Royal Society of London* 1515–1527.

Coyle, J.T. and Duman, R.S. (2003) Finding the intracellular signaling pathways affected by mood disorder treatments. *Neuron* 38: 157–160.

Davis, K.L., Kahn, R.S., Ko, G., and Davidson, M. (1991) Dopamine in schizophrenia: a review and reconceptualization. *American Journal of Psychiatry* 148: 1474–1486.

Ditto, W.L. and Pecora, L.M. (1993) Mastering chaos. *Scientific American* 8: 25–32.

Edelman, G.M. (1987) *Neural Darwinism: The Theory of Neuronal Group Selection.* New York: Basic Books.

Erikson, E.H. (1963) *Childhood and Society.* New York: W.W. Norton.

Fairbairn, R.D. (1944) "Endopsychic structure considered in terms of object relationships", in *An Object–Relationships Theory of the Personality.* New York: Basic Books, pp. 82–136.

Feinberg, I. and Guazzelli, M. (1999) Schizophrenia – a disorder of the corollary discharge systems that integrate the motor systems of thought with the sensory systems of consciousness. *British Journal of Psychiatry* 174: 196–204.

Fogg-Waberski, J. and Waberski, W. (2000) Electroconvulsive therapy: clinical science vs. controversial perceptions. *Connecticut Medicine* 64: 335–337.

Frances, A.J. and Egger, H.I. (1999) Whither psychiatric diagnosis. *The Australian and New Zealand Journal of Psychiatry* 33: 161–165.

Freud, A. (1936) *The Ego and the Mechanisms of Defence.* New York: International Universities Press.

Freud, S. (1900) "The interpretation of dreams," *Standard Edition* 4–5: 1–625.

Freud, S. (1915a) "Instincts and their vicissitudes", in *Standard Edition* 14: 117–140.

Freud, S. (1915b) "Repression", *Standard Edition* 14: 141–158.

Freud, S. (1915c) "the unconscious", *Standard Edition* 14: 159–215.

Freud, S. (1923) "The infantile genital organization (An interpolation into the theory of sexuality)," *Standard Edition* 19: 141–145.

Freud, S. (1926 [1925]) "Inhibitions, symptoms and anxiety," *Standard Edition* 20: 75–172.

Freud, S. (1938) "Splitting of the ego in the process of defense," *Standard Edition* 23: 275–278.

Freud, S. (1953–1966) *Standard Edition of the Complete Psychological Works of Sigmund Freud*, Vol. 1. London: Hogarth Press. First published 1900.

Freud, S. (1966) "Project for a scientific psychology," in J. Strachey (ed.) *Standard Edition of the Complete Psychological Works of Sigmund Freud*, Vol. I. London: Hogarth Press, pp. 295–387.

Friston, K.J. and Frith, C.D. (1995) Schizophrenia a disconnection syndrome?, *Clinical Neuroscience* 3: 89–97.

Frith, C.D., Friston, K.J., Liddle, P.F., and Frackowiak, R.S.J. (1991) Willed action and the prefrontal cortex in man: a study with PET. *Proceedings of the Royal Society of London* 244(B): 141–146.

Fromm, E. (1941) *Escape From Freedom*. New York: Rinehart.

Fuster, J.M. (1995) *Memory in the Cerebral Cortex. An Empirical Approach to Neural Networks in the Human and Nonhuman Primate*. London, and Cambridge, MA: The MIT Press.

Fuster, J.M. (1997) Network memory. *Trends in Neuroscience* 20: 451–459.

Glantz, L.A. and Lewis, D.A. (1997) Reduction of synaptophysin immunoreactivity in the prefrontal cortex of subjects with schizophrenia. Regional and diagnostic specificity. *Archives of General Psychiatry* 54: 943–952.

Globus, G. (1992) Toward a noncomputational cognitive neuroscience. *Journal of Cognitive Neuroscience* 4: 299–310.

Goff, D.C., Leahy, L., Berman, I., Posever, T., Herz, L., Leon, A.C., Johnson, S.A., and Lynch, G. (2001) A placebo-controlled pilot study of the ampakine CX516 added to clozapine in schizophrenia. *Journal of Clinical Psychopharmacology* 21: 484–487.

Goldman-Rakic, P.S. (1987) "Circuitry of prefrontal cortex and the regulation of behavior by representational knowledge," in P.F. Mountcasel and V. Bethesda (eds) *Handbook of Physiology, Vol 5*. New York: American Physiological Society, pp. 373–417.

Goldman-Rakic, P.S. (1994) Working memory dysfunction in schizophrenia. *Journal of Neuropsychiatry* 6(4): 348–356.

Goldman-Rakic, P.S. (1996) The Prefrontal Landscape: Implications of Functional Architecture for Understanding Human Mentation and the Central Executive. *Philosophical Transactions of the Royal Society of London* 1444–1451.

Gombos, Z., Spiller, A., Cottrell, G.A., Racine, R.J., and McIntyre Burnham, W. (1999) Mossy fiber sprouting induced by repeated electroconvulsive shock seizures. *Brain Research* 844: 28–33.

Grace, A.A. (1991) Phasic versus tonic dopamine release and the modulation of dopamine system responsivity: a hypothesis for the etiology of schizophrenia. *Neuroscience* 41: 1–24.

Gross, M., Slater, E., and Roth, M. (1954) *Clinical Psychiatry*. London: Macmillan.

Hallett, M. (2000) Transcranial magnetic stimulation and the human brain. *Nature* 406 (6792): 147–150.

Hartmann, H. (1939) *Ego Psychology and the Problem of Adaptation*. New York: International Universities Press, 1958.

Hartmann, H. (1950) Comments on the psychoanalytic theory of the ego. *Psychoanalytic Study of the Child* 5: 74–96.

Hartmann, H. (1964) *Essays on Ego Psychology*. New York: International Universities Press. Available online at http://en.wikipedia.org/.

Hartmann, H., Kris, E., and Loewenstein, R.M. (1964) *Papers on Psychoanalytic Psychology*. New York: International Universities Press.

Hebb, D.O. (1949) *The Organization of Behavior*. New York: John Wiley & Sons.

Herz, J., Krogh, A., and Richard, G.P. (1991) *Introduction to the Theory of Neural Computation*. Santa Fe, Santa Fe Institute: Addison Wesley.

Hinton, G.E. (1981) "Implementing semantic networks in parallel hardware", in *Parallel Models of Associative Memory*. Hillsdale, NJ: Erlbaum.

Hoffman, R.E. (1992) Attractor neural networks and psychotic disorders. *Psychiatric Annals* 22: 119–124.

Hoffman, R.E., Oats, E., Hafner, J., and Husting, H.H. (1994) Semantic organization of hallucinated "Voices" in schizophrenia. *American Journal of Psychiatry* 151: 1229–1230.

Hoffman, R.E., Buchsbaum, M.S., and Jensen, R.V. (1996) Dimensional complexity of EEG waveforms in neuroleptic-free schizophrenic patients and normal control subjects. *Journal of Neuropsychiatry* 4: 436–441.

Hoffman, R.E., Hawkins, K.A., Gueorguiera, R., Boutros, N.N., Rachid, F., Carroll, K., and Krystal, J.H. (2003) Transcranial magnetic stimulation of left temporoparietal cortex and medication resistant auditory hallucinations. *Archives of General Psychiatry* 60: 49–56.

Hokfelt, T., Bartfai, T., and Bloom, F. (2003) Neuropeptides: opportunities for drug discovery. *Lancet Neurology* 2: 463–472.

Hopfield, J.J. (1982) Neural networks and physical systems with emergent collective computational abilities. *Proceedings of the National Academy of Sciences* 79: 2554–2558.

Hwang, L.L. and Dun, N.J. (1999) Serotonin modulates synaptic transmission in immature rat ventrolateral medulla neurons in vitro. *Neuroscience* 91: 959–970.

Isaacs, S. (1952) "On the nature and function of phantasy," in M. Klein, P. Heimann, S. Isaacs, and J. Riviere (eds) *Developments in Psychoanalysis*, pp. 67–121. (Reprinted from *International Journal of Psychoanalysis* 29 (1948): 73–97.)

Jackson, J.H. (1969) Certain points in the study and classification of diseases of the nervous system. *Lancet* 1(307): 344–379.

Jo, J.H., Park, E.J., Lee, J.K., Jung, M.W., and Lee, C.J. (2001) Lipopolysaccharide inhibits induction of long-term potentiation and depression in the rat hippocampal CA1 area. *European Journal of Pharmacology* 422: 69–76.

Jung, C.G. (1954) *The Development of Personality*. New York: Pantheon Books.

Kandel, E.R. (1989) Genes, nerve cells, and the remembrance of things past. *Journal of Neuropsychiatry and Clinical Neuroscience* 1: 103–125.

Kandel, E.R. (1991) *Principles of Neural Science*, ed. E.R. Kandel, J.H. Schwartz, and T.M. Jessell. Norwalk, CT: Appleton & Lange.

Kauffman, S.A. (1993) *The Origin of Order: Self-organization and Selection in Evolution*. New York: Oxford University Press, pp. 181–218.

Kendell, R. and Jablensky, A. (2003) Distinguishing between the validity and utility of psychiatric diagnoses. *American Journal of Psychiatry* 160: 4–12.

Kernberg, O.F. (1978) *Object-relations Theory and Clinical Psychoanalysis*. New York: J. Aronson.

King, C.C. (1991) Fractal and chaotic dynamics in nervous systems. *Progress in Neurobiology* 36: 279–308.

Klaas, E.S., Baldeweg, T., and Friston, J.K. (2006) Synaptic plasticity and disconnection in schizophrenia. *Biological Psychiatry* 59: 929–939.

Klein, E., Kreinin, I., Chistyakov, A., Koren, D., Mecz, L., Marmur, S., Ben-Shachar, D., and Feinsod, M. (1999) Therapeutic efficacy of right prefrontal slow repetitive transcranial magnetic stimulation in major depression: a double-blind controlled study. *Archives of General Psychiatry* 56: 315–320.

Klein, M. (1952) "Some theoretical conclusions regarding the emotional life of the infant," in *Envy and Gratitude and Other Works, 1946–1963*. London: Hogarth Press, 1975, pp. 61–93.

Klein, M. (1958) "On the development of mental functioning," in *Envy and Gratitude and Other Works, 1946–1963*. London: Hogarth Press, 1975, pp. 236–246.

Klimesch, W., Savseng, P., and Gerloff, C. (2003) Enhancing cognitive performance with repeated transcranial magnetic stimulation at human individual alpha frequency. *European Journal of Neuroscience* 17: 1129–1133.

Klosterkotter, J. (1992) The meaning of basic symptoms for the development of schizophrenic psychoses. *Neurology Psychiatry and Brain Research* 1: 30–41.

Kohut, H. (1971) *The Analysis of the Self: A Systematic Approach to Psychoanalytic Treatment of Narcissistic Personality Disorders*. Madison, WI: International Universities Press.

Kondratyev, A., Sahibzada, N., and Gale, K. (2001) Electroconvulsive shock exposure prevents neuronal apoptosis after kainic acid-evoked status epilepticus. Brain research. *Molecular Brain Research* 91: 1–13.

Koukkou, M., Lehmann, D., Wackermann, J., Dvorak, I., and Henggeler, B. (1993) Dimensional complexity of EEG brain mechanisms in untreated schizophrenia. *Journal of Biological Psychiatry* 33: 397–407.

Koukkou, M., Federspiel, A., Braker, E., Hug, C., Kleinlogel, H., Merlo, M.C., and Lehmann, D. (2000) An EEG approach to the neurodevelopmental hypothesis of schizophrenia studying schizophrenics, normal controls and adolescents. *Journal of Psychiatric Research* 34: 57–73.

Kukekov, V.G., Laywell, E.D., Suslov, O., Davies, K., Scheffler, B., Thomas, L.B., O'Brien, T.F., Kusakabe, M., and Steindler, D.A. (1999) Multipotent stem/progenitor cells with similar properties arise from two neurogenic regions of adult human brain. *Experimental Neurology* 156: 333–344.

Kupfer, D.J., First, B.B., and Regier, D.A. (2005) *A Research Agenda for DSM-V*. Washington, DC: The American Psychiatric Association.

Laifenfeld, D., Klein, E., and Ben-Shachar, D. (2002) Norepinephrine alters the expression of genes involved in neuronal sprouting and differentiation: relevance for major depression and antidepressant mechanisms. *Journal of Neurochemistry* 83: 1054–1064.

Lamont, S.R., Paulls, A., and Stewart, C.A. (2001) Repeated electroconvulsive stimulation, but not antidepressant drugs induces mossy fibre sprouting in the rat hippocampus. *Brain Research* 893: 53–58.

Leff, J. (1987) "A model of schizophrenic vulnerability to environmental factors," in H.G.W. Hafner and W. Janzarik (eds), *Search for the Causes of Schizophrenia*. Berlin, Heidelberg, New York, Tokyo: Springer.

Lewis, D.A. (1995) Neural circuitry of the prefrontal cortex in schizophrenia. *Archives of General Psychiatry* 52: 269–273.

Lewis, D.A., Pierri, J.N., Volk, D.W., Melchitzky, D.S., and Woo, T.W. (1999) Altered GABA neurotransmission and prefrontal cortical dysfunction in schizophrenia. *Biological Psychiatry* 46: 616–626.

Liddle, P.F. (1987) Schizophrenia syndromes cognitive performance and neurological dysfunction. *Psychological Medicine* 17: 49–57.

Lotto, B., Upton, L., Price, D.J., and Gaspar, P. (1999) Serotonin receptor activation enhances neurite outgrowth of thalamic neurones in rodents. *Neuroscience Letters* 269: 87–90.

Lynch, G. and Gall, C.M. (2006) Ampakines and the threefold path to cognitive enhancement. *Trends in Neuroscience* 29: 554–562.

Magarinos, A.M., Deslandes, A., and McEwen, B.S. (1999) Effects of antidepressants and benzodiazepine treatments on the dendritic structure of CA3 pyramidal neurons after chronic stress. *European Journal of Pharmacology* 371: 113–122.

Makeig, S., Bell, A.J., Jung, T.P., and Sejnowski, T.J. (1996) *Independent Component Analysis of Electroencephalographic Data*. Cambridge: The MIT Press.

Manji, H.K., Quiroz, J.A., Sporn, J., Payne, J.L., Denicoff, K.A., Gray, N., Zarate, C.A. Jr., and Charney, D.S. (2003) Enhancing neuronal plasticity and cellular resilience to develop novel, improved therapeutics for difficult-to-treat depression. *Biological Psychiatry* 53: 707–742.

Manschreck, T.C., Maher, B.A., and Milavetz, J.J. (1988) Semantic priming in thought-disordered schizophrenic patients. *Schizophrenia Research*. 1: 61–66.

Marenco, S., Egan, M.F., Goldberg, T.E., Knable, M.B., McClure, R.K., Winterer, G., and Weinberger, D.R. (2002) Preliminary experience with an ampakine (CX516) as a single agent for the treatment of schizophrenia: a case series. *Schizophrenia Research* 57: 221–226.

Mazer, C., Muneyyirci, J., Taheny, K., Raio, N., Borella, A., and Whitaker-Azmitia, P. (1997) Serotonin depletion during synaptogenesis leads to decreased synaptic density and learning deficits in the adult rat: a possible model of neurodevelopmental disorders with cognitive deficits. *Brain Research* 760: 68–73.

McCarthy, G., Puce, A., and Goldman-Rakic, P. (1996) Activation of human prefrontal cortex during spatial and non-spatial working memory tasks measured by functional MRI. *Cerebral Cortex* 6: 600–611.

McGuire, P.K., Silberwiak, R.S.J., and Frith C.D. (1995) Abnormal perception of inner speech: a physiological basis for auditory hallucinations. *Lancet* 346, 596–600.

McGuire, P.K., Syed, G.M.S., and Murray, R.M. (1993) Increased blood flow in Broca's area during auditory hallucinations in schizophrenia. *Lancet* 342: 703–706.

Merzenich, M.M. and Kaas, J.H. (1982) Reorganization of mammalian somatosensory cortex following peripheral nerve injury. *Trends in Neuroscience* 5: 434–436.

Mesulam, M. (1998) From sensation to cognition. *Brain* 121: 1013–1052.

Meynert, T. (1968) *Psychiatry*. New York: Hafner. First published 1885.

Michael, C. (1986) *Object Relations and Self Psychology: An Introduction*. Monterey, CA: Brooks Cole.

Neely, J.H. (1991) "Semantic priming effects in visual word recognition: a selective review of current findings and theories," in D.B.G.W. Humphrey (ed.) *Basic Progresses in Reading and Visual Word Recognition*. London, and Hillsdale, NJ: Erlbaum.

Norman, R.M.G., Malla, A.K., Williamson, P.C., Morrison-Stewart, S.L., Helmes, E., and Cortese, L. (1997) EEG coherence and syndromes in schizophrenia. *British Journal of Psychiatry* 170: 411–415.

Paulus, M.P., Perry W., and Braff, D.L. (1999) The nonlinear, complex sequential organization of behavior in schizophrenic patients: neurocognitive strategies and clinical correlations. *Biological Psychiatry* 46: 662–670.

Peled, A. (1999) Multiple constraint organization in the brain: a theory for serious mental disorders. *Brain Research Bulletin* 49: 245–250.

Peled, A. (2004) *Brain Dynamics and Mental Disorders*. Tel-Aviv: Yozmot Heliger.

Perecman, E. (1987) *The Frontal Lobes Revisited*. New York: The IRBN Press.

Pertaub, D.P., Slater, M., and Barker, C. (2001) An experiment on fear of public speaking in virtual reality. *Studies in Health Technology and Informatics* 81: 372–378.

Piaget, J. (1962) The stages of intellectual development of the child. *Bulletin of Meninger Clinic* 26: 120.

Pridmore, S. and Belmaker, R. (1999) Transcranial magnetic stimulation in the treatment of psychiatric disorders. *Psychiatry and Clinical Neurosciences* 53: 541–548.

Prigogine, I. and Stengers, I. (1984) *Order Out of Chaos*. New York: Bantam Books.

Rapaport, D. (1967a [1951]) "The autonomy of ego," in M. Gill (ed.) *The Collected Papers of David Rapaport*. New York: Basic Books, pp. 357–367.

Rapaport, D. (1967b [1958]) "The theory of ego autonomy: a generalization," in M. Gill (ed.) *The Collected Papers of David Rapaport*. New York: Basic Books, pp. 722–744.

Riggio, S. (n.d.) Nonconvulsive status in clinical decision making. Available at http://appneurology.com/showArticle.jhtml?articleId=181500816.

Rizzo, A.A. and Buckwalter, J.G. (1997) The status of virtual reality for the cognitive rehabilitation of persons with neurological disorders and acquired brain injury. *Studies in Health Technology and Informatics* 39: 22–33.

Rogers, C.R. (1965) *Client Centered Therapy, its Current Practice Implications and Theory*. Boston: Houghton Mifflin.

Roland P.E. (1993) *Brain Activation*. Stockholm, Sweden: Wily-Liss Inc.

Rothbaum, B.O., Hodges, L., Smith, S., Lee, J.H., and Price, L. (2000) A controlled study of virtual reality exposure therapy for the fear of flying. *Journal of Consulting and Clinical Psychology* 68: 1020–1026.

Rumelhart, D.E. and McClelland, J.L. (1986) *Parallel Distributed Processing: Exploration in the Microstructure of Cognition*, PDP Research Group edn, Vols 1 and 2. Cambridge, MA: The MIT Press.

Sadock, B.J. and Sadock, V.A. (eds) (2004) *Kaplan and Sadock's Comprehensive Textbook of Psychiatry*, 8th edn. Philadelphia, PA: Lippincott Williams & Wilkins.

Saito, N., Kuginuki, T., Yagyu, T., Kinoshita, T., Koenig, T., Pascual-Marqui, R.D., Kochi, K., Wackermann, J., and Lehmann, D. (1998) Global, regional, and local measures of complexity of multichannel electroencephalography in acute, neuroleptic-naive, first-break schizophrenics. *Biological Psychiatry* 43: 794–802.

Selemon, L.D., Rajkowska, G., and Goldman-Rakic, P.S. (1995) Abnormally high neuronal density in the schizophrenic cortex: a morphometric analysis of prefrontal area 9 and occipital area 17. *Archives of General Psychiatry* 52: 805–818.

Singer, W. (1995) Development and plasticity of cortical processing architectures. *Science* 270: 758–764.

Snyder, S.H. (1976) The dopamine hypothesis of schizophrenia: focus on the dopamine receptor. *American Journal of Psychiatry* 133: 197–202.

Soares, J.C. and Innis, R.B. (1999) Neurochemical brain imaging investigations of schizophrenia. *Biological Psychiatry* 46: 600–615.

Spitzer, M., Braum, U., Hermle, L., and Maier, S. (1993) Associative semantic network dysfunction in thought-disordered schizophrenic patients: direct evidence from indirect semantic priming. *Biological Psychiatry* 34: 864–877.

Stanley, J.A., Williamson, P.C., Drost, D.J., Carr, T.J., and Tompson R.T. (1995) An in vivo study of the prefrontal cortex of schizophrenic patients at different stages of illness via phosphorus magnetic resonance spectroscopy. *Archives of General Psychiatry* 52: 399–406.

Sullivan, H.S. (1953) *The Interpersonal Theory of Psychiatry*. New York: Norton.

Thompson, K., Sergejew, A., and Kulkarni, J. (2000) Estrogen affects cognition in women with psychosis. *Psychiatry Research* 94: 201–209.

Tononi, G. and Edelman, G.M. (2000) Schizophrenia and the mechanisms of conscious integration. *Brain Research Reviews* 31: 391–400.

Tononi, G., Sporns, O., and Edelman, G.M. (1994) A measure for brain complexity: relating functional segregation and integration in the nervous system. *Proceedings of the National Academy of Sciences* 91: 5033–5037.

Tononi, G., Sporns, O., and Edelman, G.M. (1996) Complexity measure for selective matching of signals by the brain. *Proceedings of the National Academy of Sciences* 93: 3422–3427.

Van-Praag, H.M. (1997) The future of biological psychiatry. *CNS Spectrums* 2: 18–25.

Vincelli, F., Choi, Y.H., Molinari, E., Wiederhold, B.K., and Riva, G. (2001) A VR-based multicomponent treatment for panic disorders with agoraphobia. *Studies in Health Technologies Informatics* 81: 544–550.

Weinberger, D.R. (1987) Implications of normal brain development for the pathogenesis of schizophrenia. *Archives of General Psychiatry* 44: 660–669.

Wernicke, K. (1881) *Text Book of Cerebral Diseases*. Berlin: Karger.

Wickliffe, A.C. and Warren, T.P. (1997) Metaplasticity: a new vista across the field of synaptic plasticity. *Progress in Neurobiology*, 52: 303–323.

Winn, P. (1994) Schizophrenia research moves to the prefrontal cortex. *TINS* 17: 265–268.

Xian, H.Q. and Gottlieb, D.I. (2001) Peering into early neurogenesis with embryonic stem cells. *Trends Neuroscience* 24: 685–686.

Yurgelun-Todd, D.A., Renshaw, P.F., and Cohen, B.M. (1995) Functional MRI of schizophrenics and normal controls during word production. *Schizophrenia Research* 15: 104–110.

Index

Page numbers in *italics* refer to figures.

Printed and bound by CPI Group (UK) Ltd, Croydon, CR0 4YY

01/11/2024

01782626-0006